Dr Daniel Golshevsky

Dr Golly is a Melbourne-based paediatrician and father of three.

Specialising in unsettled babies and poor sleep (inspired by his three beautiful yet highly unsettled babies), Dr Golly has developed his philosophy through his work with thousands of babies over nearly two decades of practice. Knowing there's no one-size-fits-all solution, Dr Golly aims to turn up the volume on parents' innate instincts to maximise their understanding of their baby's cues.

Many jokingly refer to him as a 'baby whisperer', but he likes to think of himself more as a 'parent whisperer' – cheering you on to be the most empowered, confident parent he knows you can be.

Whether you've seen him in a clinic, read this book or completed his online programs; he wants all parents to rest assured that there is no better parent for their babies than them!

Background and education:
- Bachelor of Medicine, University of Melbourne
- Fellow of the Royal Australasian College of Physicians
- Former Chief Resident Medical Officer of The Royal Children's Hospital, Melbourne

Proud:
- Red Nose Australia Ambassador
- Clinical Perinatal Mental Health Champion of PANDA
- Professional Member of the Australian Breastfeeding Association
- Peer-reviewed author on paediatric sleep and obesity
- International clinical practice guidelines reviewer
- General paediatric trainee lecturer

 Follow Dr Golly on socials @drgolly

  Learn more about his sleep programs and podcast drgolly.com

YOUR
BABY
doesn't come with a
BOOK

To my greatest teachers: my wife, my parents
and my three remarkable children.

– Dr Golly

Hardie Grant acknowledges the Traditional Owners of the Country on which
we work, the Wurundjeri People of the Kulin Nation and the Gadigal People
of the Eora Nation, and recognises their continuing connection to the land,
waters and culture. We pay our respects to their Elders past and present.

Hardie Grant Children's Publishing
Wurundjeri Country
Ground Floor, Building 1, 658 Church Street
Richmond, Victoria 3121, Australia
www.hardiegrantchildrens.com

ISBN: 9781761212888
First published 2023

Image credits: *page 56* dwphotos/Shutterstock, Inc *page 57* ©K Reeder
Photography 2023, Nelly B/Shutterstock, Inc *page 58* Karen Culp/Shutterstock,
Inc *page 59* Akkalak Aiempradit/Shutterstock, Inc *page 120* Daniel Golshevsky
page 143, 144 all reproduced with permission from ©DermNet 2023 *page 145*
reproduced with permission from ©DermNet 2023, Soft Light/Shutterstock, Inc
page 146 Aisylu Ahmadieva/Shutterstock, Inc *page 151* 2p2play/Shutterstock,
Inc, Ruth Jenkinson/Science Photo Library, spass/Shutterstock, Inc

A catalogue record for this
book is available from the
National Library of Australia

Printed in China by Leo Paper Group

FSC
www.fsc.org
MIX
Paper from
responsible sources
FSC® C020056

The paper this book is
printed on is certified against
the Forest Stewardship
Council® Standards and
other sources. FSC®
promotes environmentally
responsible, socially
beneficial and economically viable
management of the world's forests.

Publisher Marisa Pintado
Cover design Kelly Elphick
Internal design Chris Forsyth
and Hannah Schubert
Editorial Penelope White with
Vanessa Lanaway and Emma Schwarz
Production Amanda Shaw
Illustrator Cora Muccitelli

24531

YOUR BABY
doesn't come with a
BOOK

Dr Daniel Golshevsky

PAEDIATRICIAN

Hardie Grant

BOOKS

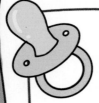

Contents

Birth-day and beyond

The first four weeks of parenthood

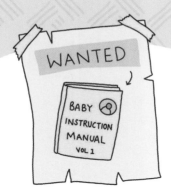

Introduction

I'm Dr Golly, paediatrician and father of three.

Congratulations on the birth – or imminent arrival – of your little bundle of joy. These gorgeous little munchkins carry with them all **our love, our hopes, our emotions** – but, unfortunately, they **don't carry an instruction manual.**

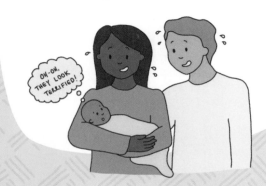

I see hundreds of unsettled babies every year, and have also had the pleasure of three gorgeous, yet terribly unsettled, babies of my own.

I've been encouraged countless times over the years to write a book about the newborn period, but have resisted because there is no one-size-fits-all approach.

Each baby needs different things at different ages and developmental stages. So instead of trying to force a baby into a mould, this book is designed to **empower you**, as parents and caregivers, to:

1. know what to expect in the first four weeks

2. better understand your baby

3. interpret their cues

4. respond accordingly.

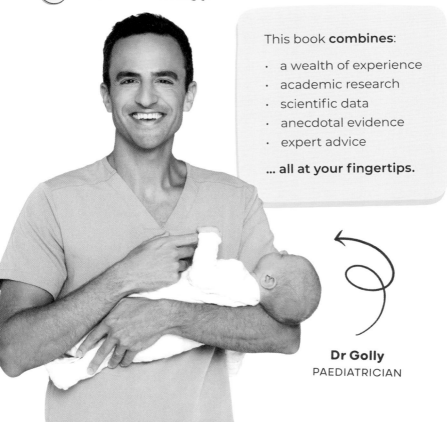

This book **combines**:

- a wealth of experience
- academic research
- scientific data
- anecdotal evidence
- expert advice

... all at your fingertips.

Dr Golly
PAEDIATRICIAN

The first four weeks after a newborn's arrival are an exciting, adrenaline-filled challenge.

It's sad that sometimes we perceive it as something to be *survived*.

There are dozens of ways to prepare for life with a newborn and **build the foundations for you and your baby to settle into a nice rhythm.**

Getting your baby into a steady rhythm in the first few weeks of life will help **establish a consistent schedule and has long-term benefits for the whole family.** It'll help your family be happy and enjoy the unequivocal benefits of good sleep.

Why long-term? Because we know that parents of unsettled babies report sleep problems persisting well beyond the age of five years!

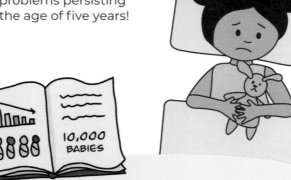

An Australian study of more than 10,000 babies found that for a third of those who experienced poor sleep as newborns, those sleep problems got worse as they got older. They also lacked self-regulation, which is a crucial skill to help maintain and focus attention, and control emotions and behaviours.

The study suggests benefits not just for your sleep and wellbeing as parents, but also for **the long-term emotional health and wellbeing of your child.**

Some people refer to the early newborn phase as the fourth trimester.

The concept of the fourth trimester comes from the evolution of our frontal lobe. This is what separates us from apes and other mammals.

The frontal lobe is where we house the CEO of our brain, and it's what enables our executive functions.

Humans may be the most intelligent of animals because of our frontal lobes, but the size of our brains means that human foetuses have to arrive 'earlier than planned' just so that they can exit a pregnant woman's pelvis.

So babies are born relatively early, exceptionally dependent, and physically quite unimpressive!

This means babies require almost constant attention, frequent feeding and for virtually everything to be performed for them.

Although physically unimpressive, babies are by no means emotionally or cognitively mediocre. Babies are not poor communicators who cry as their only means of language. Quite the opposite, in fact! Babies are far more intelligent than we give them credit for – we just need to decipher what they are communicating to us.

I am going to teach you:

- what's normal and what's abnormal
- what your baby is capable of and when they need to be given more time to develop these capabilities
- to realistically plan for life with a newborn.

I will **dispel the many myths that exist** and empower you to **harness the fantastic parenting instincts that you already possess.**

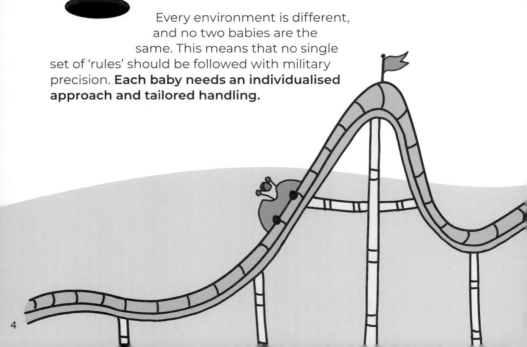

There's no one-size-fits-all solution

Say it with me again – there is no one-size-fits-all solution when it comes to babies and parenting.

A baby sits at the centre of concentric rings of family, culture, community and society. **Every culture is different, every child is different.** There are infinite variables influencing the way you raise your child.

It is absurd to think that the incredibly complex relationship between baby and parent can be reduced to an instruction manual.

Every environment is different, and no two babies are the same. This means that no single set of 'rules' should be followed with military precision. **Each baby needs an individualised approach and tailored handling.**

In addition to being a paediatrician, I've trained in infant mental health and worked with sleep specialists, lactation consultants, parentcraft/maternal health nurses and sleep schools.

I've read all the books, studied all the journals and watched all the videos.

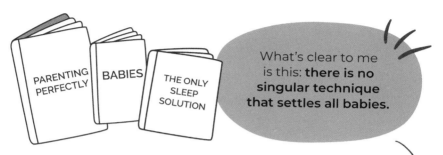

PARENTING PERFECTLY

BABIES

THE ONLY SLEEP SOLUTION

What's clear to me is this: **there is no singular technique that settles all babies.**

If you're looking for a rigid routine or settling technique, you won't find it here.

Instead, my philosophy is to find the solution that's right for your baby and right for your parenting style.

Use this resource to learn how to communicate with your baby. This will help you understand their cues, confidently respond to their needs and create secure attachment, while thoroughly enjoying this *roller-coaster* we call parenthood.

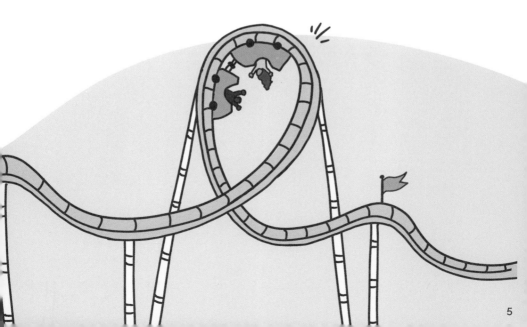

Babies drink more than milk

Contrary to what many people believe, babies are excellent communicators.

It is we adults who complicate communication with things like sarcasm, nuance, exaggeration and dramatic gestures.

You see, **babies drink more than just milk.**

Babies are phenomenally sensitive.
Just as an animal can sense fear, so can
a baby sense anxiety or worry.

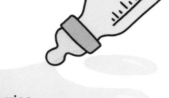

Babies drink your emotions, your worries and your fears. When a nervous adult holds a baby, they carry tension through their biceps – right where the baby often rests their head. This tension transfers directly to the baby, and they will be less likely to settle as a result.

If you are empowered to understand
your baby, interpret their cues and signs
correctly and respond accordingly, then
you'll ooze confidence. And your baby will
guzzle that down, along with their milk.

anxious

stressed

calm

loving

They will drink your love, confidence and infatuation – your desire to care and protect.

happy

This works in a cycle. The more empowered
you are, the more confident you are.
The more confident you are, the
more relaxed you feel. The more
relaxed you feel, the more settled
your baby will be. The more
settled your baby is, the more
confident you are ... and so
the cycle happily continues!

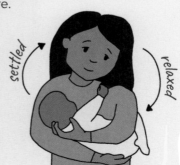

Turning the volume up on your parental instincts

Instinct is a fascinating thing.

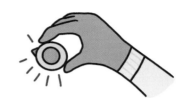

The Oxford Dictionary describes **instinct** as an innate pattern of behaviour.

Parental instinct is the innate pattern that ensures the survival and development of our offspring. This already exists in us all.

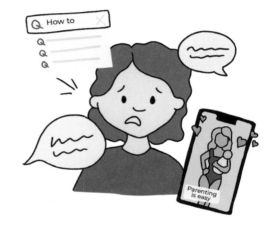

You don't need to download it, activate it or update it.

It's the voice inside you, what some people refer to as their sixth sense or gut feeling. It's always there, but in our modern society, the volume is often turned right down, or sometimes it's even muted entirely. Excessive noise, selectively curated social media feeds, uncontrolled online content and unsolicited advice from family, friends or strangers all serve to sow doubt and fuel anxiety.

If we learn to understand our offspring better, we gain confidence and turn up the volume on our parental instinct. Then the parent–baby relationship becomes a true **two-way conversation**, and the early steps of parenthood are filled with joy, not dread.

Secure attachment

Paediatrician Dr William Sears promoted the concept of **attachment parenting** in the 1950s. This refers to fostering a strong relationship between parent and child through physical closeness and empathy.

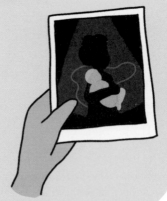

In the weeks following birth, **babies should be close to their caregiver as much as possible,** as though their umbilical cord is still attached. In these first weeks, you cannot 'over-love' a baby.

While attachment parenting is crucial and beautiful, it is not always easy to achieve. What good is a parent to a child if that parent is:

- overwhelmed?
- exhausted?
- under-slept?

Parental empathy and responsiveness require a parent to be:

- present
- happy
- well rested
- not anxious

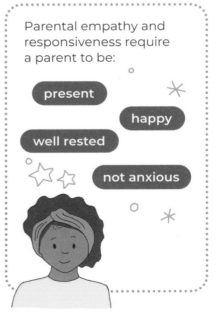

That's why, in 1991, psychologists Ainsworth and Bowlby pioneered the concept of **secure attachment** in children. This is more than just attachment. **It's the foundation for good long-term social and emotional outcomes** – everything we want for our children. Secure attachment is achieved through the presence of a **consistently available parent**, who is attuned to their child's needs and emotions.

This means the newborn period is not just about feeding, clothing and protecting the child – **it's also about protecting the parents**, and helping the child to build resilience and learn to self-settle when developmentally appropriate.

To be available, that parent must also prioritise their own wellbeing. This includes:

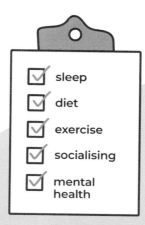

- ☑ sleep
- ☑ diet
- ☑ exercise
- ☑ socialising
- ☑ mental health

The power of dads and non-breastfeeding parents

Never underestimate the unique and powerful potential of the non-breastfeeding parent.

Babies arrive into families of all different shapes and sizes. From couples to single parents, blended families, adoptive parents and more. It's wonderful that almost everyone has the ability to become a parent nowadays.

But regardless of the look of the family unit, it's important that we take a moment to focus on the role of the non-breastfeeding parent. For simplicity, I'll just refer to them as the father for now, but know that this can refer to anyone else in the home.

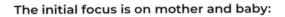

The initial focus is on mother and baby:

When a baby enters a family unit, the focus is usually on the baby and on the mother, especially if the mother is breastfeeding. This makes perfect sense – the baby is the new arrival, requiring round-the-clock care and attention, and the mother is recovering from pregnancy and delivery, while also being the key source of the baby's nutrition.

But I'd like to shift the paradigm a little, and **put the spotlight on fathers**.

Fathers play a significantly greater role than many people think. In fact, we might just be the key to having a well-settled baby and entire family unit.

To understand why fathers can be the key, let's first learn what happens in the mother's brain following the birth of her baby ...

Oxytocin is a hormone that rises significantly in mothers following childbirth. Sometimes described as a drug of love, oxytocin plays a fundamental role in social bonding, love, trust and generosity.

Oxytocin has also been shown to activate and grow a part of the brain called the amygdala. The amygdala is important for processing memory, and drives emotions like fear, anxiety and aggression.

The heightened amygdala activation after childbirth is what drives a mother's hypersensitivity to their baby, making her attentive, loving and deeply affectionate.

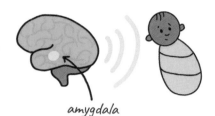

amygdala

But this also makes the mother far more likely to want to feed an unsettled baby.

When a breastfeeding mother picks up her crying baby, it's close to impossible to avoid feeding. The baby is being held right next to a food source, knowing that they will be comforted by proximity and the sucking reflex – so they are very unlikely to settle for anything less from their mum! And the mother's body and hormones are responding to the baby's distress.

That is why fathers are more likely to be able to resettle a baby, if something wakes them before a feed is due. **Fathers don't have that same oxytocin surge. Fathers also don't smell of breastmilk.**

So when fathers hold a crying baby, we send them a very clear message – through our touch, through our hormones, through our energy – that they are not going to get fed. Babies – astute communicators – can sense this and are far more likely to settle down.

This is why fathers can be much more successful at settling babies than mothers.

We can use this to our benefit when we're trying to establish a nice routine, or resettle a baby who has woken unexpectedly early.

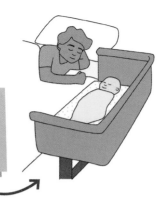

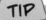 **TIP**

Whenever possible, have baby sleep on dad's side of the bed, so they're not overly stimulated by mum's proximity.

Fathers can do anything for their baby; the only thing they can't do is breastfeed. Having fathers more involved has many benefits:

- They extend far beyond just establishing a good routine (although this is a pretty good one!).
- More involved fathers have significantly lower levels of paternal postnatal depression and anxiety.
- When having a second or third child, having fathers perform the bulk of the care of a newborn frees up the mother to spend more quality time with the older siblings. This prevents predictable, major behavioural challenges in 2–4-year-olds, who miss being the centre of attention when a new baby arrives.
- And last, but most incredibly, when fathers assume a greater role in parenting, or are the main caregiver, they too develop higher levels of oxytocin and have the same amygdala response.

If your baby wakes early:

Have dad make the first attempt at resettling. Not only does this improve the likelihood of achieving the sleeping/feeding rhythm, but it also enables mothers to sleep more, speeding up recovery from childbirth, boosting breastmilk supply and replenishing energy stores.

Late-evening feeds:

Fathers can take over the late-evening feed if they want to be involved in the feeding process too. This can be achieved with expressed breastmilk and a bottle, or with formula.

Note: If you're working on establishing breastfeeding, avoid this in the first month.

What to do when dad's not home?

Mums ask me all the time what they're meant to do if dad's not home, or away for work.

The best thing you can do is put on one of dad's hoodies. This masks the smell of breastmilk and makes the baby think it's dad coming to resettle them.

Milk-free zone

A note to all dads and non-breastfeeding parents:

This oxytocin surge is not limited to mothers. It's not childbirth that brings it on; it's just being close to a newborn. It's settling a cry, changing a nappy, striving for that reciprocal smile. Giving love to this little bundle is what opens up this well of unconditional love and emotion.

For years, women have been reaching greater levels of achievement in education and work – but with no equivalent reduction in the expectation that they will do the majority of newborn parenting.

Workplaces are starting to wake up to this inequity and we're seeing more companies offer elongated paternity leave packages (we'll talk more about this next). This is the seismic societal shift we need in order for fathers to be more involved in the care of newborns – bringing immeasurable benefits for the baby, undoubtable benefits for the mother, and infinite benefits for us dads.

13

Protecting a breastfeeding mother

This is core to my philosophy as a paediatrician.

When you're thinking about your postpartum plans, protecting both the breastfeeding mother and the newborn are the two greatest priorities for a family.

priority #1
priority #

THE ONLY THING YOU *CAN'T* DO TO SUPPORT A BREASTFEEDING MOTHER IS BREASTFEED.

More often than not, a breastfeeding mother has many challenges to work through, even for those who take to breastfeeding well. These can include producing the right amount of milk, mastering your newborn's latch, monitoring engorgement, keeping nipples damage-free, avoiding or dealing with mastitis – all while recovering from childbirth!

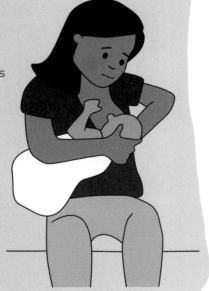

We'll talk about this concept more throughout the book, but when in doubt …

Protect these breastfeeding women with every resource you have.

DR GOLLY
PHILOSOPHY

Beyond this book

This book is designed to give you the foundational tools and confidence to:

- understand your baby better
- interpret their signs and cries
- hone your parenting skills
- empower you as parents to trust your innate parental instincts.

You'll notice there are no routines in this book – I don't recommend introducing them until your baby is six weeks old (when they are roughly 5–6 kilograms). In the first six weeks, you are just getting to know each other, and if you're breastfeeding, you'll be working on establishing supply. In Part 3, we'll discuss sleep cycles and finding your rhythm in the first four weeks.

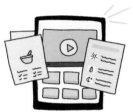

Beyond this book, the accompanying online Dr Golly Sleep Programs will help you introduce routines and settling techniques that suit your family. My aim here is to help you understand what your baby is capable of at every developmental stage.

So, what is your baby capable of?

With the removal of hurdles:

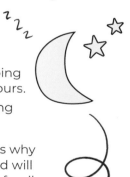

- by six weeks, most babies are capable of sleeping through the night; that is, for seven straight hours.
- by six months, most babies are capable of going a full 12 hours overnight between feeds.

My online programs will help you identify reasons why your baby may not be reaching those targets, and will suggest tweaks you can make to get your whole family sleeping through the night (if that's what you want).

Sleep, development and nutritional demands change over the course of childhood, so our programs change too, evolving with your child, up to five years of age.

The ultimate aim of my book and programs is to have **empowered families** – and **sleeping babies.**

> The first few days and first four weeks can be
> an adrenaline-charged, hormone-filled roller-coaster,
> so a little planning can make a big difference.

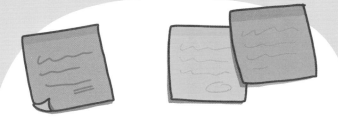

Before the baby comes: *postpartum planning*

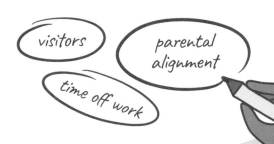

Parental leave

When it comes to planning your parental leave, there's no right or wrong answer, and many decisions are based on job security and finances. Feel confident that whatever choice you make, you're making the best decision for *your* family at this time.

Parental leave expectations change based on:

· culture
· employer
· socioeconomic realities.

· ·

When my first baby arrived, I worked solely in the public health system and was afforded two days' leave before returning to night shift in the emergency department. It was brutal, but it was the reality of my situation and I had little control over it.

· ·

Non-birthing parental leave

More and more government and workplace policies are updating parental leave plans to include fathers too – and to give non-birthing parents access to extended parental policies. This is amazing and the seismic societal shift many have yearned for.

Many workplaces now offer a period of leave, to be taken by either parent, at any time, within the first 12 months of a baby's arrival.

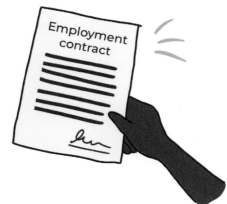

Some non-birthing parents will choose to take off one or two days a week over an extended period of time. This can certainly be helpful, but there are other alternatives that may be more beneficial.

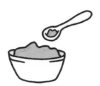

If it's achievable, it is incredibly special and valuable for both parents to have the first month together.

That said, it's also worth considering other options:

- Think about delaying paternity leave until your baby is well established on solids (in the latter half of their first year of life), particularly if the birthing parent wants to transition back to work.

- Consider taking on primary parental duties (taking into consideration a family's plans for ongoing breastfeeding).

  This can be:

1. Good for your relationship

Until you take on the role of primary carer, you can never appreciate the full extent of the workload; the physical and emotional challenges involved.

2. Good for the child

Having both parents spend intense periods of time with a baby or child is incredibly beneficial for parental bonding, as well as demonstrating to older siblings the new models of family functioning.

3. Good for you

You'll get a hit of oxytocin – see page 11 for more on the hormonal changes and love that arise in non-breastfeeding parents who take on intense childcare duties.

4. Good for workplace equality

The idea that a male employee is equally likely to take extended paid leave means that any employer bias (perceived or otherwise) is spread across all genders.

Managing visitors at home

Whether you're the birthing or non-birthing parent, the focus in the weeks and months after birth is on bonding with your new baby, getting to know each other, and adjusting to life as a parent. Yet – understandably – your baby's arrival can cause much excitement among friends and family, all of whom may want to visit immediately!

> Protecting your home may seem an unusual manoeuvre – and some of this advice may seem oppositional or difficult to enact – but any friend, family or colleague who has children will immediately understand. Don't feel the need to justify yourselves.

The newborn period can be incredibly isolating, particularly when we no longer live with our 'village'. For this reason, I encourage visitors and socialisation at every desired opportunity.

However, I think we should reconsider how we visit families with newborns, and make sure it's all about making their lives easier.

This section is actually not for you – it's more relevant for your friends and family! But the more we discuss this period as a society, the easier the newborn period will be for all families.

Tip 1:
Visitors should make your life easier, not harder

In many cultures, the fourth trimester is seen as a period when the breastfeeding mother is treated like a queen, and friends and family wait on her hand and foot.

While for many active mums this may seem intolerable, it can be helpful to consider the first month postpartum to be a long period of recovery.

Confinement may not be your thing, but your recovery, establishing breastmilk supply and bonding with the baby (for both parents) should be the priorities.

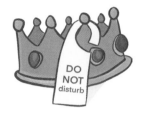

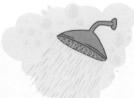

Tip 2:
You don't need a perfect house

You don't need to 'host'.
You can be in your tracksuit or pyjamas ALL DAY LONG.

You don't need to prepare food or drinks – quite the opposite, in fact: your visitors should do this for you.

If the house is messy and you haven't showered, the first thing visitors can do is start cleaning, look after baby and send you to enjoy a long shower or a walk outside.

Tip 3:
Visitors should arrive with food

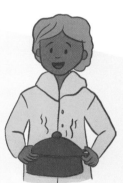

If people are coming for a visit around mealtimes, they should bring the food!

If they are popping in for coffee, ask them to pick one up on the way.

Fresh, wholesome, easy-to-eat food is ideal. Lots of people bring things for the freezer, but sometimes a freshly prepared salad is all new parents want!

Tip 4:
Leave an esky/cooler at the front door

If you're worried about people just 'popping in' and don't want unannounced visitors, put a sign on the front door that says something like: 'Baby and mother are sleeping, please leave any food in the esky, and text that you dropped in. Thank you!'

Tip 5:
There's nothing wrong with visitors helping while they're there

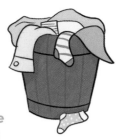

When they arrive, your ideal visitors will assess what needs doing and get to work! They can watch the baby while you have a shower, do a load of washing, empty the nappy bin, cook dinner, pick up the groceries ... anything that takes a job off your list is perfect.

Another great idea is for visitors to text a list of items and have the parents pick two. Some ideas:

· watch the baby for an hour
· do a load of washing
· fold washing
· clean a room
· cook dinner, etc.

Tip 6:
Allow time and space for breastfeeding

In my opinion, if someone criticises a mother for breastfeeding in public, they should be arrested! There is no purer act on earth than breastfeeding, and no place where it should be deemed inappropriate.

That doesn't mean all women feed confidently in a crowd, and certainly some mothers may not want people watching and/or giving unsolicited feedback. If you prefer feeding at home, time your outings accordingly, ensuring you leave plenty of time to get home for feeds.

Run your own race here, and trust your instincts about what feels right for you and your baby.

Tip 7:

If the baby needs to sleep – let them sleep

While it's fine to wake your baby to prevent them oversleeping or to establish a routine, you should never feel like you need to wake your baby so that someone can have a cuddle or a photo. Doing that means the visitor leaves with a photo while you're left with an unsettled, overtired baby.

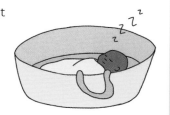

Tip 8:

If you're not ready for visitors, that's okay!

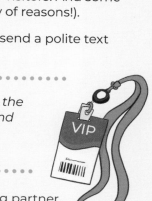

While I recommend socialisation for your own health and wellbeing, sometimes the timing won't be right and you may not feel up to having any visitors. And some visitors you may not want at all (for a variety of reasons!).

If this is the case, you or your partner could send a polite text along the lines of:

* *

Thank you for all the lovely wishes! We're in the thick of the post-birth recovery right now and not quite up for visitors – we'll let you know when we are.

* *

If you're the non-birthing, non-breastfeeding partner, it's YOUR job to manage who gets to spend time with your VIPs as they learn to breastfeed and recover together. Take over the texts and calls whenever you can.

Managing visitors and illness

With regard to viral exposure, my approach is simple and straightforward – people shouldn't visit you and your newborn if they're symptomatic. Really, this goes for visiting anyone, and attending work too.

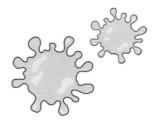

Newborns are vulnerable due to their young age and developing immune systems. However, this does not mean they need to be cocooned in their homes for fear of viral exposure. Many parents elect to remain home until their baby's first round of immunisations (after leaving the hospital). This is not necessary and not advised. Immunisations have a cumulative effect, meaning one dose does not provide complete protection.

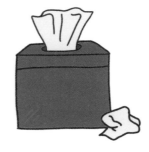

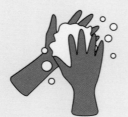

Common sense prevails, just as it has since Hungarian physician Ignaz Semmelweis first discovered that washing his hands between patients dramatically reduced hospital death rates back in the 19th century. Ask visitors to be well before they arrive, or when you catch up generally.

Visitors and vaccinations

I recommend a whooping cough (pertussis) vaccine booster for anyone spending a lot of time with a newborn, if they have not had a booster in the last ten years. Immunity to pertussis wanes over time, and pertussis is particularly dangerous for young babies.

If you and your family feel strongly about certain vaccines, you have every right to make your own choices. I urge open, courteous conversations around this topic, with a particular focus on a happy, settled baby and recovering mother.

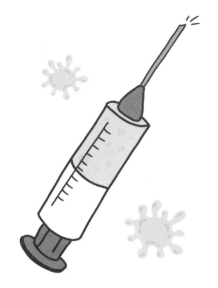

TIP

An easy way to manage this is to send a group text message to friends and family, blaming me!

Hi loved ones, we can't wait to welcome our new baby to the world shortly. We'd love you to come for a cuddle, and our paediatrician has recommended that visitors have their whooping cough vax booster updated if more than ten years old. Also, just as a general rule: delay your visit if you've got a cold. Thanks so much!

Gifting

When it comes to gifting, depending on culture and circumstance, there will no doubt be a few family members or friends who are keen to purchase a gift for you and/or your baby. This is a beautiful gesture, generous and thoughtful. My advice is to have a list of all the helpful items that people may consider gifting you.

Don't be afraid to do the following:

- When someone asks what they can get you, send them a list of items you want or need.

- Ask people to purchase practical things, like a digital thermometer or a white noise machine.

- Explain that certain gifts need to align with your core values. For example, gender-neutral clothing, limited plastic products, recycled or second-hand toys, etc.

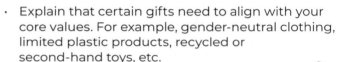

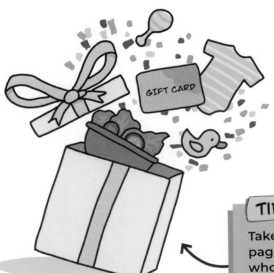

In my experience, people love knowing that they are getting you something you need/want and will use.

TIP

Take a picture of these two pages and send it to anyone who asks what to get you!

'Doing' gifts

'Doing gifts' are incredibly powerful for new parents! These might be things like:

- **meals** – a home-cooked meal is great, as are food delivery vouchers, or food trains (this is where different friends/ family each take a night of the week to cook for you … so you don't end up with 472 lasagnes in the freezer)

- **babysitting**

- **lactation consultant voucher**

- **cleaning** – offering to clean or paying for a cleaning service is one of the most valuable gifts you can give new parents

- **washing**

- **grocery shopping.**

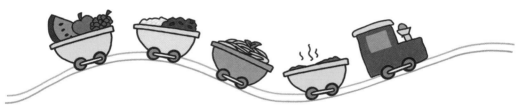

Flowers

In my experience, flowers sent to the hospital are beautiful and generous, but often challenging. I frequently see fathers trying to juggle a suitcase, car seat and vases when leaving the hospital. Often, flowers will be left in the room.

For many families, the day they leave the hospital will be the first time they've put a newborn into a car seat, so minimising the fuss and extra items can be advantageous. My advice would be to politely ask for some of the 'doing gifts' mentioned above, rather than flowers.

Where your baby will sleep

The nursery

Before their baby arrives, many parents have this idea of a perfect nursery of a whimsical place with gorgeous natural light, a bassinet with cute teddies and cosy blankets, a sweet mobile hanging overhead and a rocking chair in the corner for feeding.

What many parents quickly discover is that:

- the baby sleeps in your room

- when it comes to sleep, darkness is your friend

- SIDS (Sudden Infant Death Syndrome) guidelines advise removing all toys from cots

- when they're lying in the bassinet, you want your baby to be sleeping, not being stimulated by a mobile.

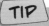

TIP

Hang the mobile over the nappy change table to keep them distracted/entertained while changing.

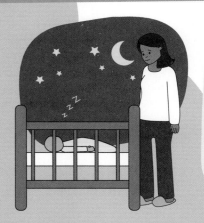

When trying to pick a room in the house for the nursery, the quietest and darkest room is ideal. Temperature regulation (hot and cold) is also highly preferable.

Room-sharing

I always strongly recommend that the bassinet be on the non-breastfeeding parent's side of the bed.

We'll talk in depth about the ideal sleeping conditions for babies and safe sleep guidelines in the upcoming chapters. Note: the Red Nose Foundation recommends room-sharing for the first 6–12 months.

Babies are incredibly noisy sleepers, and these sounds often wake parents, though the child is still sleeping peacefully. Moving the cot to the dad's or non-breastfeeding parent's side of the bed, or to the end of the bed, can be helpful, as this means your baby is less likely to smell breastmilk, or be woken by parents' movements and sounds.

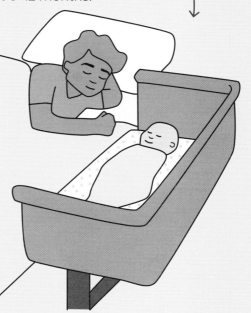

What do I need to buy?

Many parents ask me what they need in the newborn phase, and my answer is always the same: *not as much as you think!*

Big-ticket items

 A bassinet or cot that's small enough to fit beside your bed.

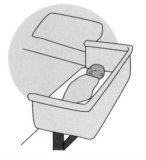

 A carrier. Our babies love being close to us, and they also love being upright. Many parents find themselves marooned if their baby will only sleep on them; a carrier keeps your hands free and means you're able to walk around while still keeping your baby close to you.

 A pram. It's even better if there's a breathable bassinet, so your baby can lie flat and sleep safely on the go. And make sure it will fit in the boot of your car!

Get the rain and sun covers that fit the pram so you're not at the mercy of the elements.

 TIP

Practise getting the pram up and down and packed away into the car well before your baby arrives, so you won't be flustered when you have to do this with a newborn.

4. **Car seat.** Allow time to have this properly fitted by a trained professional before the baby is due.

5. **A play mat for tummy time.** Washable is my number-one tip with these!

6. **Change table.** They don't have to be whizz-bang; these days you can just buy attachments or baskets that sit on top of drawers or tables. The main thing is to protect your back, and make sure you're not bending over beds, etc. You'll find as your baby grows, you'll want something pretty sturdy.

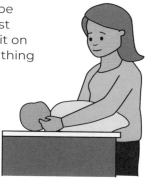

7. **Somewhere to bath the baby.** You can do this in a normal bath, but lots of families love a plastic bath on the bench. Just make sure there's a drain nearby so you're not lugging heavy water around – and be mindful of your back if you need to bend over a larger bathtub.

8. **Nappy bin.** In the middle of the night, you don't want to be going outside to dispose of dirty nappies.

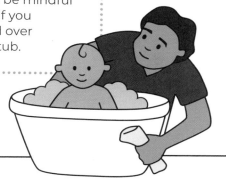

Nitty-gritty items

 Nappies

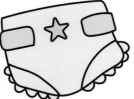

- Disposable or cloth – it's up to you. I see a lot of families doing a mixture of both.

- There are thankfully more sustainable disposable options these days; there are also cloth nappy services that will launder them for you, or disposable inserts that can be put into structured cloth nappies.

- Make your purchases high volume and low frequency if possible! Just remember: babies grow fast, so you'll progress through sizes rapidly.

- Be sure to donate unused nappies to local charities or friends with babies on the way.

 Onesies (cotton with zips, not buttons)

Tip: Get the ones with feet and hand covers; then you don't need to worry about socks and mittens, which are potential choking hazards.

- Use zips whenever possible; just watch out for fingers, toes and skin. Always keep your finger underneath the connecting sides when moving the zip, to protect the baby. Buttons are fiddly and noisy, and often wake babies at the worst possible time.

- Remember, this isn't a fashion parade. Newborns spend nearly all their time sleeping, burping or feeding. This means that soft, simple outfits are what you need. If fancy outfits are your thing, save them for when your baby is a bit older.

3. **Swaddles.** Large cotton/jersey wraps are best as they have a bit more stretch.

See page 131 for swaddling techniques.

4.

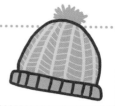

A beanie for colder climates.

5.

Face washers – you can never have too many!

6. **Old-fashioned nappy cloths or cloth wipes.** They are incredibly handy to clean spills, put over your shoulder, under bottoms etc. Trust me, you'll find many uses for them!

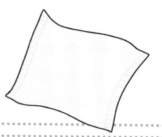

7. **White noise source.** There are many free apps available that create these sounds; portable USB charged machines for sleeping on the run and plug-in machines for the house. See page 123 for more on white noise.

8. **Block-out blinds.** There are many block-out blinds available for purchase, including temporary ones that stick onto the window glass.

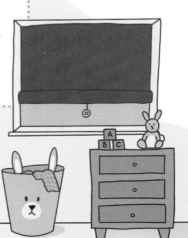

Medical items

1. **Thermometer.** A non-touch option is best for newborns. Any fever in the first months of life should be reviewed by your local doctor.

2. **Cotton-wool balls.** Soak them in warm boiled water and wipe your baby's eyes if they get gunky or crusty. This helps to milk the tear ducts and clear any blockage.

3. **Nappy cream.** Learn to apply this liberally, and invest in plenty! Zinc is the active barrier, the other ingredients are not as important.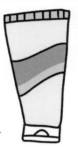

4. **Saline nose spray or drops**. The salty water is used to alleviate nasal congestion (often used in conjunction with the snot-sucker).

5. **Snot-sucker** – a device to literally suck out nasal congestion. This is one of the yuckiest and most satisfying things you'll do as a parent. Trust me, your dismay upon reading this will rapidly evaporate after the first suction. These things are magic.

6. **Baby nail clippers.** In the first four weeks the nails should just 'peel off' if they get too long, but there are some terrific options once trimming is required. Keep your baby's nails short, so they don't scratch their face (or yours).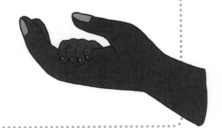

Feeding items

1. **Breast pump**, if applicable. You can usually hire these in the early weeks and months from your hospital or local breastfeeding support group, so you can wait to see if you need one.

2. **Bottles with teats.** Even if you plan to exclusively breastfeed, I still recommend offering a bottle of expressed breastmilk at least 2–3 times a week to avoid bottle rejection (once milk supply is established).

3. **Breastmilk freezer storage bags.** Write the expressed date **before** filling!

4. **Nipple cream**

5. **Nipple shields and healing covers**, if required.

6. **Formula.** Note: this should be avoided in the first four weeks of your baby's life if you're trying to establish breastmilk supply (see page 70 on supply and demand, and page 94 on breastmilk and formula for more). However, I find most families relax more if there's a 'third breast' in the cupboard on standby.

7. **Sterilisation equipment.** You can sterilise bottles in a pot on the stove, but sterilisers are affordable, incredibly efficient and safe to use.

8. **Dummy.** You may or may not need one (there are many pros and cons, which we'll discuss on page 119).

Postpartum care items for mum

1. **Maternity pads**

2. **Perineal ice packs.** These will sit on top of the maternity pad and help with both pain and inflammation.

3. **Pain relief**

4. **Postpartum high-waisted underwear** (compression and cotton)

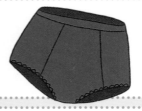

5. **Postpartum compression leggings or bike shorts**. These are to repair abdominal muscle separation after birth. Compression wear provides support through your perineum, caesarean scar or both, and corrects your posture, all while helping your body feel more supported after birth. Compression tights can help with any lower limb swelling which can be common for some women post-birth.

6. **Appointments with a lactation consultant.** These magicians can greatly improve the breastfeeding experience for mother and baby, and are worth the investment.

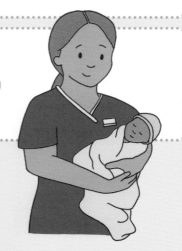

Hospital/birthing bag

Don't pack the kitchen sink; keep it minimal and simple. You'll find that everything you really need is readily available at the hospital.

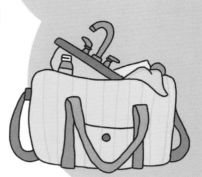

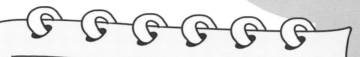

- ☑ Nappies, onesies and swaddles for baby
- ☑ Birthing clothes for mum
- ☑ Post-birth comfy and compression clothes for mum
- ☑ Post-birth high-waisted, comfy and compression underwear for mum
- ☑ Toiletries for mum (and maternity pads if your hospital doesn't supply them)
- ☑ Drink bottle (ideally one that you can open with one hand)
- ☑ Overnight bag/toiletries for partner, if they're staying
- ☑ Phone charger! An extra-long charging cord is a bonus.

Birth plans

There are entire books, training courses and healthcare departments dedicated to this topic – it's by no means my area of speciality.

What I do know is that **a trauma-free birth (where possible) leads to much better outcomes for both baby and mother**.

· ·

My top tips for birth plans are:

1. Be empowered

- This might be through a hospital-led course, an at-home consultation, a book or an online program. Whatever your preferred choice is, get in and learn about the birthing process (together).

- Understand the different interventions: what they are, when you may need them and when it's safe and okay to say no to them.

- Yes, giving birth is one of the most natural things out there, but it's important to understand the process of labour – what can go right, what can go wrong – and how the hospital or birthing centre will deal with you. The more you know about what to expect, the stronger you'll be as a birthing team.

2. Be flexible

- Many families I talk to have this ideal scenario of a calm, holistic, intervention-free vaginal birth. But the reality is, you often don't get a choice about what happens, and you'll ultimately do whatever is safest for both mother and baby.

- Your ability to have an open mind about what's to come will be a very powerful thing.

- For many mothers, this may be one of the few times in your life when you have zero control over a situation, and that can be incredibly daunting. Remember, control the bits you can, and be open and flexible to what will eventuate.

3. If you're the non-birthing partner, be the patient advocate

- Dads and partners, it's your job
to make sure your partner has
everything she needs. Be it a water
bottle, the lights dimmed, a gym
ball to sit on, the TENS machine turned up
or taken off, the midwife to be told she's
too chatty or that the anaesthetist needs to
hurry – whatever it is, it's your job to advocate on
her behalf. You are her voice, her advocate, her cheerleader.

4. If you're not aligned with what's happening, speak up early

- Whether it's your midwife, obstetrician, partner or the
temperature of the room, if something is making you
uncomfortable, speak up early. In my experience, if you're
not aligned with your healthcare provider or the institution,
this is where things can go really wrong.

- Open, honest and courteous communication will lead to
better outcomes for all.

5. Don't think of pain relief as failure

- This is a really hot-button topic, but I think lots of women
need to hear this: if you need/want an epidural or other forms
of pain relief, you're not a failure. An intervention-free birth
may be the goal for many, but pain relief may be needed.
Don't let pride get in the way of asking for it.

> The ultimate goal is a happy and healthy mother
> and baby. Do whatever you need to achieve this,
> and be open to the idea that it won't always go
> smoothly – and it definitely won't be like the movies!

Postpartum planning and prioritisation

Families often have an intricate birth plan and a perfect nursery, but not the faintest idea what to do with a baby when it arrives home. Don't worry. Even as a paediatrician, I was this parent once.

If you're reading this book, you're on the right track!

A postpartum plan is literally planning for the period after birth; it can encompass anything and everything you'll need to thrive, not just survive, with your new baby.

Things in your postpartum plan could be:

1. Being open to a vaginal or caesarean recovery.

It might seem odd that this is the first item on the list, but most families rightly assume they'll have an uncomplicated vaginal birth; sometimes that's not possible. Being open to the mental and physical recovery from any type of birth is important.

2. If either parent has had anxiety or depression previously, creating a postpartum mental health plan.

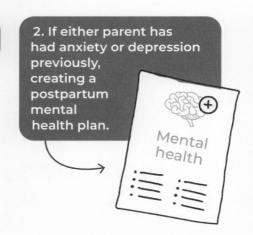

Mental health

3. Having a clear understanding of budgets and financial planning.

Many families drop to one income in the year after having a baby and this can be tough. Finances are one of the biggest concerns for many growing families.

Budget plans

4. Getting on a waitlist for childcare if that's what your family wants/needs.

5. Planning parental leave.

Having two weeks together at the start is what I strongly recommend. The first four weeks together is ideal, but a luxury very few families can manage.

6. If a non-breastfeeding parent is planning to take extended parental leave, having a plan for bottles is really important.

I see so much stress and anxiety caused by bottle rejection, so it's important to be thinking about this from day one. Whether it's formula or breastmilk, babies will be drinking milk until they're at least 12 months old.

Bottle acceptance

7. Lining up help for the first weeks after birth. This could be:

- weekly or fortnightly cleaners

- a lactation consultant ready to go

- prepared meals

- grocery shopping pre-ordered

- babysitters, so you can have some time out to reconnect.

Planning how you want to parent (together)

The key to secure attachment is **conscious parenting**, ensuring your child feels safe, seen, soothed and secure.

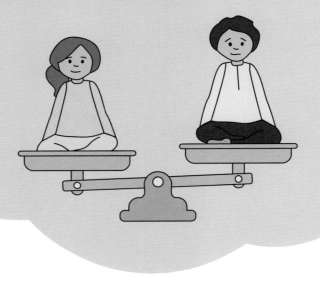

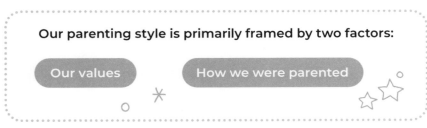

Our parenting style is primarily framed by two factors:

Our values   How we were parented

Remember, **our values are subjective** – they're not consciously chosen, but typically shaped by deep beliefs we adopted from our parents (though these may change over time). They reflect what we think is important, both for ourselves and for others around us.

Prior to a child's arrival, talk openly with your partner about the type of parents you want to become and what your parental values are.

Agenda

- What about your childhood do you want to replicate?

- What about your own upbringing would you like to avoid in your own parenting?

- Identify areas where you differ with your partner and try to find a middle ground. Parental alignment and consistency from caregivers is what children yearn for.

- Remember that different parenting styles needn't be a source of stress for parents, but rather an opportunity to learn from one another and bolster your parenting skills.

TIP

Pass this book to your partner if they're nearby and get them to read this section. Then plan a time to chat about this when you've both had time to reflect.

Try to avoid shaming your own parents. They were probably doing the best they could with the information and resources they had access to at the time.

Parental alignment

Being aligned as parents is paramount when raising children.

When both caregivers **give a child a consistent message**, it helps them to learn what is expected and how to react. It also minimises parental conflict, which is a frequent reality when managing high-stress situations, particularly while experiencing sleep deprivation.

Tips for couple alignment:

- If you're reading a book (like this), completing a program or even just researching different ideas, make sure both caregivers complete the coursework or read the information. If there's *only one* partner doing this, your parenting alignment can become imbalanced very quickly. This is relevant for birth and beyond – you never stop learning as parents.
- If it's possible, complete research or courses together! This way you can discuss topics while they are fresh. Both parents should be empowered with all the information, and one should never be made to feel that they're being 'lectured' by the other.
- Once a week, have a 'parent planning night'. It's not terribly romantic, but it may be beneficial for your relationship and general family harmony.

Parenting is the most intricate team sport there is. By aligning your strategy, respecting each other's views, engaging in reading, research or content and always being open to discussions or new ideas and planning together, you'll find that both your parenting and your relationship will be stronger.

The need for parental alignment will become more apparent as your baby grows. This conversation is continuous; it will evolve as you grow together as both parents and as partners.

Planning to leave the house

In the first four weeks, a lot of families will choose to bunker down at home, spend time together and let visitors come to them. This is absolutely fine!

Whether the birthing mother is recovering from a vaginal or caesarean birth, she will need rest.

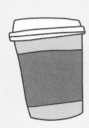

Vigorous activity will never be recommended by your obstetrician or midwife. However, you might want to venture out for a short stroll for some fresh air, or walk to get coffee – this is great too!

I recommend starting small and close by, and building your confidence – and listening to your body. Don't let your first outing be a wedding with 300 people – you wouldn't believe how many times this happens!

Getting out of the house is important for your physical and mental health. As discussed, newborns are incredibly docile and will usually sleep anywhere, so a trip in the pram or carrier for a sleep will rarely be a concern.

Pre-kids

Post-kids

If you're going further than 'nearby', remember to leave the house with everything you need:

- nappies
- wipes
- spare clothes for you and the baby

- if breastfeeding, wear an outfit you can feed in
- if bottle-feeding, bottles, formula and water

Couple strategies

Before your baby arrives, discuss the labour split in the household. A non-exhaustive list of some things to talk about include:

- ☑ cooking
- ☑ cleaning
- ☑ tidying/packing away
- ☑ washing (as well as folding and packing away washing)
- ☑ late-night feeds
- ☑ night-time settling/resettling
- ☑ changing nappies
- ☑ emptying nappy bins
- ☑ grocery shopping
- ☑ general shopping: baby stuff, birthday gifts, etc.
- ☑ meal planning
- ☑ bill paying
- ☑ financial planning
- ☑ travel planning and booking
- ☑ daycare enrolments
- ☑ post-birth government paperwork
- ☑ doctor's appointments/maternal health nurse check-ups
- ☑ family diary management.

There's often the assumption that the primary carer will take on the majority of this list, 'because they're home anyway'. While that can be okay in some families, in others it can cause burnout and resentment. Looking after a baby is a full-time job, especially in the early weeks!

If you have the resources or friends/family who want to help, outsource some of these tasks.

It's really important to:

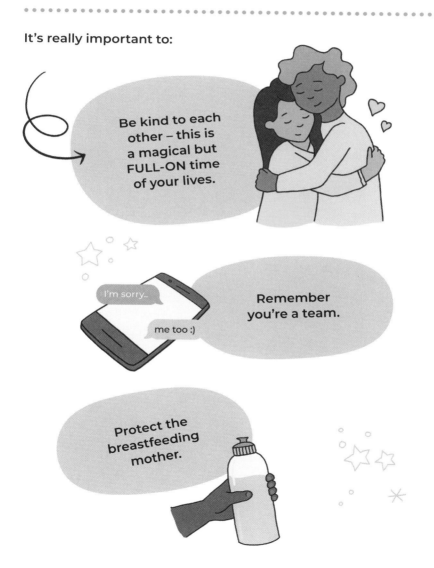

Be kind to each other – this is a magical but FULL-ON time of your lives.

I'm sorry..

me too :)

Remember you're a team.

Protect the breastfeeding mother.

It's crucial that parents of newborns seek help when needed and make life as simple for themselves as possible, especially in the first few months of their baby's life. **Go back to basics, and try to slow life down where you can.**

Some strategies include:

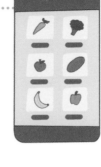

- Do your grocery shopping online.

- Use meal delivery services if available.

- Plan your meals and calendarise important tasks/events/dates.

- Ask for help from a relative, friend or neighbour.

- Take shifts overnight if possible, while one parent goes to bed early. If your baby settles early, ensure you both head to bed too.

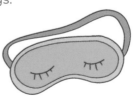

- Get out for some fresh air and a walk every day.

- Invite a friend over for a coffee if you don't feel up to going out.

- Remember it's okay to say 'no' to things.

- Rest when the baby sleeps. This can be a very frustrating line to hear, but more often than not, the washing can wait, social media can wait, and, in fact **most** things can wait. You need sleep for your mental and physical health, so prioritise it.

- Engage with friends or your new parent group.

- Seek out supports if you need help or are feeling down. There's an entire chapter dedicated to mental health in the postpartum period, starting page 210.

See pg. 210

TOP TIPS for having a plan about who does what:

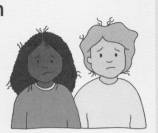

☒ Don't negotiate the plan at 3 am.

☒ Don't negotiate when there's a crying baby.

It's also important to remember how all this started.

If possible, create a space in the home where there's no newborn influence – no nappies, wipes, toys, etc. A place where you can feel like you and your partner are the only two people in the world.

With all the focus on the baby and the cumulative sleep deprivation, it's important to acknowledge that you're both doing an incredible job. Remind each other that you are participating in the most magnificent, magical and important process of your lives – moulding a child, nourishing them and sharing your love.

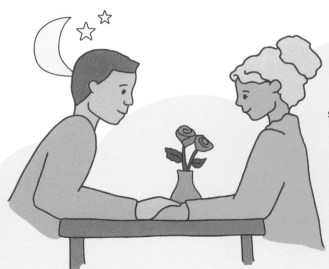

When you're spending so much time smelling dirty nappies, it's important to pause and smell the roses too.

> I want you to hold your baby for the first time knowing that this baby is the luckiest baby in the world to have you as their parent.

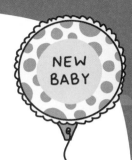

Birth-day
and beyond

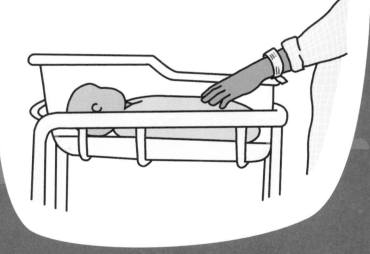

The first four weeks, and particularly the first 24–48 hours, are a magical, adrenaline-filled roller-coaster.

In the following chapters, we'll discuss hormonal changes, establishing breastfeeding, first poos, baths, swaddling, rashes ... and the fact that your baby will basically look like an alien. The great news is that newborns are pretty docile, so if you can stay calm and relaxed in the first days of your baby's life, your baby most likely will too.

While we will talk about feeding and sleep cycles, what you do need to be prepared for is feeding every three to four hours around the clock. This can seem really daunting – particularly for the breastfeeding mother, who is recovering from birth. You'll be amazed at what you can do, and empowered with all the knowledge of what to expect you will not just survive, you will thrive during this time. This is a recurring theme, but the key here is to protect the breastfeeding mother. If she's rested, fed, hydrated and feeding well during this period, this will set you all up for a lovely, positive cycle.

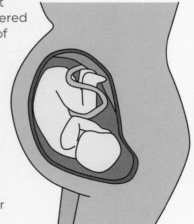

Prepare for the hours after birth

Skin-to-skin contact

For both vaginal and caesarean births, as long as your baby is well after birth, skin-to-skin contact should be started straight away, and is exceptionally important.

The benefits of skin-to-skin are incredible, calming and relaxing for both mother and baby.

According to Unicef's Baby-Friendly Initiative, skin-to-skin contact also:

· regulates the baby's heart rate and breathing
· helps them to transition more successfully to life outside the womb
· stimulates digestion and an interest in feeding
· helps regulate temperature
· allows transfer of the mother's good bacteria to the baby's skin, providing protection against infection
· stimulates the release of hormones to support breastfeeding and mothering, one of which is oxytocin (our love hormone).

Newborns who have prolonged skin-to-skin contact with their mother after birth, regardless of the mode of delivery, are more likely to breastfeed successfully. In 2020, the World Health Organization (WHO) published a study in the *British Medical Journal* which found that 90 minutes of uninterrupted skin-to-skin contact, where a baby is dried and laid directly on their mother's bare chest after birth, maximises the chance for the baby to be physically ready to breastfeed.

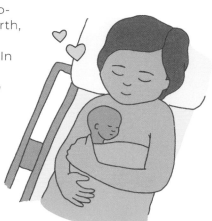

Only break this contact for the resuscitation of the baby after birth, or if mum is unwell. Even if your choice is not to breastfeed, skin-to-skin offers wonderful benefits, and should be encouraged wherever possible. Dads and other non-breastfeeding caregivers can have skin-to-skin contact too.

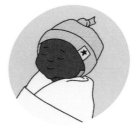

It's really important that both mother and baby stay warm. Often, the hospital staff will provide a little beanie for the baby's head, and warm blankets. This is not a fashion item; it's to ensure warmth is maintained.

Sometimes after a caesarean section, skin-to-skin contact might be briefly interrupted while your baby is weighed, measured and attended to. However, many hospitals now prioritise skin-to-skin contact as long as it's safe, so it's a good idea to ask your midwife or obstetrician if this is possible.

Baby care after birth

In the hours after birth, your midwife or paediatrician will thoroughly examine your baby from head to toe. Your baby will also have their all-important weight, length and head circumference measured and documented for you.

Post-birth care for mothers

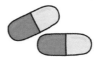

Regardless of how your baby was born, there will most likely be some pain and discomfort post-birth. It's important that the mother can move around enough to help recover from the birth, but also look after her baby. As I always say, a mother must look after herself before she can look after her baby. Any pain relief offered to a postnatal mother in hospital (or provided for her to take home) will be safe to take when breastfeeding. While minuscule amounts do transfer through to breastmilk, the benefits of taking regular pain relief (when needed) far outweigh the cons.

Competing advice in hospital

You'll have different midwives on different shifts during your hospital stay, and more often than not, depending on when they were trained and their own personal experiences, they'll have different advice about feeding/settling/bathing/everything. This can be *incredibly confusing* for new parents, who can't yet know what will work best for them or their baby. You're still learning!

Don't get flustered by this – trust your instincts about what feels right for your family. Remember, there is no single *right way* to look after a baby – every family and every baby is different. Enjoy your hospital stay, and make the most of the midwives looking after you and your baby. Take in all their advice, and use what works best for you and your family.

Managing visitors at the hospital

In many countries and across different cultures, visitors are not permitted to enter maternity wards. This is intended to protect postpartum mothers. Interestingly, visitor restrictions on maternity wards during the COVID-19 pandemic unequivocally improved early outcomes for mothers and babies, who were allowed more time and space to bond and recover from childbirth!

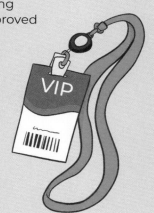

For couples, it might not be possible, or even desirable, to impose a complete ban on postpartum visitors – but remember: like any good nightclub bouncer, it's the non-breastfeeding parent's job to manage who gets to spend time with their VIPs as they learn to breastfeed and recover together.

It's normal for your baby to look a bit like an alien

What is normal? Most new parents are surprised at their baby's initial appearance. Babies never come out looking like they're ready for their first Instagram photo shoot. The more prepared you are, the less confronting this will be. It can also help to know what skin and appearance changes are normal in the first weeks of life, to avoid unnecessary worry and anxiety.

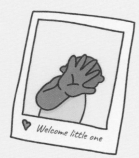

Welcome little one

Vernix

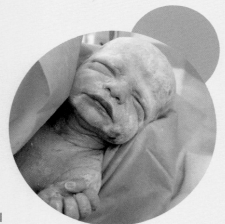

In addition to being covered in blood from the birthing process, babies can also have a white waxy coating on their skin, called vernix caseosa. While it may not look very pretty, it's best not to remove it too quickly, as it provides many benefits to the skin.

Vernix starts to appear around halfway through pregnancy and slowly disappears towards the final weeks in utero. This means that babies born early may have more vernix than those born on – or after – their due date. In addition to being the greatest moisturiser that money can't buy, vernix also lubricates the baby for an easier birth, and keeps them warm immediately afterwards.

If the vernix is not stained with meconium (baby's first bowel action), then I recommend leaving it on the skin for at least 48 hours – just in time for baby's first bath.

Head shape

Babies often appear with misshapen heads. A newborn's skull bones are soft and flexible. Instead of one skull bone, there are multiple bones that can overlap during the birthing process, intentionally reducing the baby's head diameter to help with delivery.

Following birth, these overlapping bones may be seen or felt as bumps and ridges on the baby's head. Most babies who are born headfirst have spent many weeks squashed into a very tight space, which can 'mould' the head into an oblong shape. Fluid can also collect in the part of the skull that first passes through the cervix, resulting in a 'conehead' appearance, called caput (caput succedaneum). Fluid, moulding and bumps usually resolve within the first few hours or days of life.

Umbilical cord

The umbilical cord is the baby's lifeline during pregnancy, connecting them to the placenta. Shortly after birth, the cord will be cut, leaving a short stump attached to the baby. Over the course of 1–2 weeks, this stump will dry, darken, shrivel and shrink, before detaching naturally, leaving behind your baby's brand new belly button.

During the detachment, small amounts of yellow ooze sometimes appear – there is no need to be concerned about this. However, if your baby's cord stump continues to ooze beyond two weeks, have them seen by a doctor, as treatment may be required.

Care of the cord is simple. You do not need to use soap during a bath; simply wet the area, then pat it dry with a soft towel. When putting a nappy on your baby, try to fold the nappy underneath the cord, to keep it clear of any soiling.

Although uncommon, the cord can become infected. If the belly button area becomes hot, red or tender, or if your baby develops a fever or is not feeding well, have them seen by a doctor.

Hair

Many babies are born quite hairy. This fine, dark body hair, called lanugo, is usually present for the first month of life, before falling out. Babies born with head hair may lose this in the first few weeks of life, before it starts to regrow.

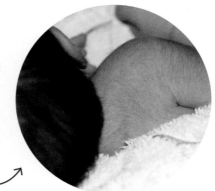

Tongue

A frenulum (Latin: *bridle*) can frequently be found throughout the human body: in both male and female genitalia, under the tongue, in the brain and in our guts. The frenulum's job is to hold a mobile organ in place, much like an anchor holds a boat. These are normal, necessary parts of the human body.

A tongue-tie – or ankyloglossia – is where the lingual frenulum (the anchor under the tongue) inserts closer to the tip of the tongue and anchors it too tightly to the floor of the mouth, limiting tongue thrust and sideways movement. Occasionally, a dent is visible in the base of the tongue, or in severe cases, the tip will appear heart-shaped. When necessary, a tongue-tie can be cut/divided by a healthcare professional.

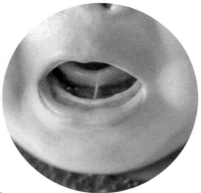

If your baby has a small tongue-tie with no heart-shaped tip and a tongue thrust that reaches to the lower lip, the tongue-tie rarely needs to be cut. Dividing a tongue-tie is not without risks, including bleeding and infection. A mild/moderate tongue-tie will not lead to speech difficulties or problems swallowing, though many parents worry that the mere presence of a tongue-tie necessitates removal.

While there is no evidence to suggest an impact on eating solids or speech, there is a documented association between severe tongue-tie and nipple pain for breastfeeding mothers. The reduced tongue movement can cause painful grazing or pinching. The challenge here is to differentiate between the pain of breastfeeding with severe tongue-tie and the natural, common discomfort that can come with breastfeeding any baby.

Not all tongue-ties cause breastfeeding issues

To painlessly, exclusively breastfeed a completely settled baby is a blessing enjoyed by few families. Often if a tongue-tie is present (even if it is very mild), it will be blamed for every feeding issue. The fact is, some babies are unsettled – for myriad reasons – and some breastfeeding mothers experience latch difficulties, discomfort, pain or other complications, and a mild tongue-tie will have nothing to do with it.

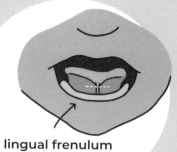

lingual frenulum

Speak with a lactation consultant if you're having breastfeeding difficulties. Identify possible causes of unsettled infant behaviour and do not be pressured into booking your baby for an expensive and potentially dangerous tongue-tie cut, if it is not justified.

Jaundice in newborns

Jaundice describes the yellowing of the skin (most visible in the whites of the eyes) that occurs in every newborn baby. This happens due to a build-up of bilirubin in the baby's skin.

To understand why this happens, consider one of the most important cells in our body – the red blood cell. This cell carries oxygen around our body, to fuel our systems. In order to ensure they are working at perfect function, we constantly refresh them, by making them and then breaking them down, in a 90-day cycle.

As with any breakdown, the waste products (bilirubin) need to be cleared by the body. A pregnant woman does this for an unborn baby, but once that cord is cut, it's now baby's job to clear this waste themselves. Babies will develop this clearance ability, but it can take a few days, which leads to the waste accumulating under the skin, driving that yellow discolouration.

> While the discolouration is harmless, if it worsens, jaundice can cause lethargy. This will make babies tired and impact their feeding.

So, while mildly jaundiced babies need no treatment, as it approaches a moderate level – these babies need to have their hydration monitored. The more a baby feeds, the faster they clear the jaundice, so parents will be encouraged to feed more often or give a volume top-up, to prevent the complications of moderate or severe jaundice.

Ultraviolet exposure can also speed up the clearance of jaundice, but we don't recommend you simply put your baby in the sun at home, because you need to expose a huge amount of skin to the UV rays, which is neither feasible, nor safe.

This is because babies can:

- be bothered by the bright light,
- get sunburnt when hot, or
- become too cold in the cooler months.

If the jaundice is moderate to severe, doctors will use a medical UV machine in hospital, which includes eye protection for babies.

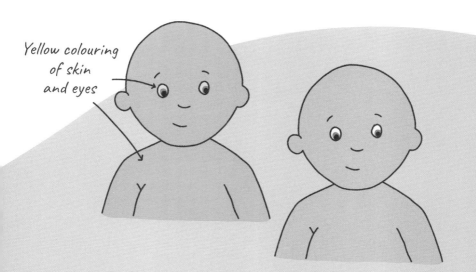

Yellow colouring
of skin
and eyes

Poo

Meconium

Many parents get a real shock when they see their baby's first poo, because it rarely looks like what they expect. It's a thick and sticky tar-like substance called meconium, usually dark green or black, and completely odourless. It usually occurs within the first 24 hours of life.

Occasionally, babies will pass this while still in utero, or during the delivery process. If your baby passes meconium before being born, there is a risk that their first breath will actually bring some of this into their lungs. Meconium is harmful to newborn lung tissue, so if your baby is born with meconium-stained waters, they will be observed closely for 1–2 days to ensure no meconium entered the lungs.

Changes in poo colour

The meconium slowly transitions to different types of poo, which can range from yellow to brown to green, and everything in between. There is a big range of normal, but this transition usually occurs within the first week of life.

Pasty light brown
Normal poo for babies having formula, a peanut butter consistency.

Mucus in poo
This poo looks snotty or like shiny string. This can indicate an intolerance to something in a breastfeeding mother's diet or the formula (we'll discuss intolerances on page 104). See your doctor if your baby has mucus in their poo.

Black
This can be a sign that your baby has ingested some blood; it is not normal. See your doctor if your baby has black poo. Sometimes it is from cracked/bleeding nipples when breastfeeding. Meconium passed in the first few days is black (very dark green) but your baby's poo should not stay black in colour.

Thick brown
Normal poo once solids begin, resembling more of an adult poo, stronger smell than when just on milk feeds.

Mustard yellow
Normal breastfed-baby poo, pasty or seedy. Breastfed babies can also have looser brown or green poo.

Red
This is not normal and could be a sign that your baby is bleeding. Can also be a sign that your baby has an intolerance. See your doctor if your baby's poo is red.

White
This is not normal. This could be a sign that the liver may not be producing enough bile, making the poo white in appearance and with a chalky texture. See your doctor.

Dark green or greenish black
Meconium passed in the first few days. This is your baby's first poo and is sticky and tar-like. It is a combination of amniotic fluid, bile and fatty acids that your baby ingested while still in the womb.

Light green
Normal formula-fed baby poo; it has simply passed through your baby's gut faster.

Frothy
We will cover in lactose overload on page 91.

When to worry about poo

We don't like to see stools that are white/pale, black (once the meconium has passed) or red; these babies need to be seen by a doctor.

Many parents have concerns regarding the frequency of their child's bowel actions, and worry their child might be constipated. When concerned about constipation, you should look at the consistency of the poo, rather than the frequency with which it is passed.

Some babies will poo with every feed, others may only poo once a week. As long as the stool is soft and easily passed, you shouldn't worry about how frequently your baby is pooing. *Breastfed babies are almost never constipated.*

Mucus or blood in the poo is a sign of intolerance (to breastmilk or formula), and should be reviewed by a doctor.

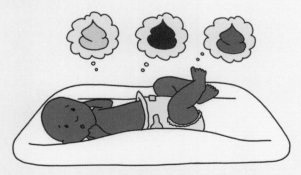

Breastfeeding and bottle-feeding

There is no room for judgement

This chapter could last forever. It is important for both birthing and non-birthing parents to read this, but there is one thing mothers need to know above all else.

You are enough.

You have conceived, nourished and grown this human, delivered them into this world and now protect them and nurtured them through their every whim. You are enough.

When the topic of milk arises, there is no room for judgement, because you are enough. Your choices are determined by culture, circumstance, health, logistics and a multitude of factors entirely out of our control. You are enough.

However you continue to feed your baby, know that you are enough and there is no room for judgement. If you'd like to further your understanding of breastmilk, formula, intolerances, associations and more, please read on. But always remember, you are enough.

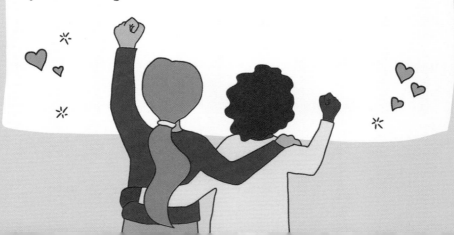

Colostrum

Colostrum is the first milk a mother will produce. It is nutrient rich, yellow in colour, and thicker than breastmilk.

Colostrum is like liquid gold for your newborn. This nutrient-dense milk is high in antibodies, necessary sugars and antioxidants. It will help build your baby's immune system, jump-start their gut function, and seed a healthy gut microbiome in the first few days of life.

Many parents are often shocked to learn that a mother starts producing colostrum before her baby is born! In the last couple of weeks leading up to the baby's due date, a midwife or obstetrician might bring up the topic of hand-expressing colostrum. This can be helpful in many ways, but is by no means essential.

Expressing colostrum prior to delivery means parents have a stored collection to use after the baby's arrival. This can be especially helpful in the setting of:

- gestational diabetes (babies can experience low blood sugar levels after birth; having colostrum on hand provides a terrific sugar supply)
- some neonatal medical conditions, such as having a cleft lip/palate, where the baby has difficulty attaching to the breast and may require feeds via specialised bottle
- some cardiac and neurological conditions (which may result in your baby's suck being less powerful).

It's always important to discuss hand-expressing with your primary pregnancy caregiver, and to remember that this should only be done later in pregnancy (36 weeks onwards) if you are considered low-risk.

Hand-expressing can be a helpful skill to master before your baby arrives, as there is so much information to learn and digest after birth. Knowing how to hand-express means there is one less thing to take in! If you are able to express colostrum, you can collect it in small syringes, which can then be stored safely in the fridge or freezer and given to your baby after birth.

Don't worry if you can't express any colostrum, or simply don't want to. Babies are the best at getting it out, and are designed to do just that. If you do hand-express before you give birth, this doesn't mean that you won't have any left for your baby – your body will simply produce more and more with ongoing stimulation and removal until your milk comes in.

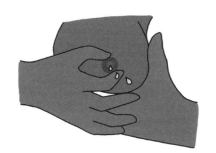

Storage of colostrum:

- room temperature for 4–6 hours if below 26°C
- fridge for 3–5 days
- freezer for 3–6 months.

Your milk will 'come in'

After colostrum, around day 3–5 after your baby is born, your milk begins to 'come in'.

During this time, your breasts will most likely feel tingly/warm/firm and occasionally hard (we'll talk about this more later).

While it's a seamless process for many, there are quite a few things that may impact or cause a delay in your milk coming in:

- birth trauma
- premature birth
- hormonal imbalances
- severe stress
- caesarean (surgical) delivery
- bleeding after birth
- infection or illness with fever
- hormonal imbalances – including thyroid conditions
- IVF or PCOS (polycystic ovarian syndrome).

How is breastmilk made?

Stimulation and removal of milk are key.

If you have delayed supply, don't be disheartened; keep stimulating and removing any colostrum and milk by breastfeeding or expressing via hand and/or hospital-grade pump until your baby is successfully breastfeeding. Listen to your midwives, doctors and lactation consultants about how to manage your baby's calorie intake.

Two key ingredients

The two key ingredients to making breastmilk are:

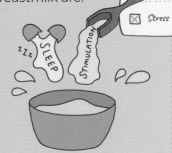

Ingredients
- ☑ Stimulation
- ☑ Sleep
- ☒ Stress

Stimulation: Breastfeeding is driven by supply and demand. That means the more a baby stimulates and effectively removes milk from the breasts by sucking, the more milk will be produced. The more often and effectively a baby breastfeeds (or milk is removed via expression) the more a mother will make.

Sleep: This is important as much of a breastfeeding mother's energy is required to make milk. During sleep, Prolactin levels increase, helping breastmilk supply grow and establish.

Stress and **fatigue** can have very detrimental effects on milk volume and flow. It is important to do everything possible to protect the breastfeeding mother.

Remember, the only thing you can't do to support a breastfeeding mother is breastfeed. Literally everything else can be done by someone else.

Breastmilk letdowns

A breastmilk letdown or drop, also known as the milk ejection reflex, is the physical process of milk being released from the breast in response to the baby's sucking or other stimuli.

> Your milk 'letdown' is controlled by two hormones:
>
> 1. **Prolactin**. This peaks 30 minutes after the feed begins, and tells your body to make more milk, in preparation for the next feed.
>
> 2. **Oxytocin**. This peaks earlier than prolactin, sometimes even as a mother merely *thinks* about feeding, or hears her baby crying (sometimes it can even be the sound of a *different* baby crying). Oxytocin causes the breast to push the milk towards the nipple and eject.

A letdown can be a different experience for different mothers and can happen at different times. Some may feel a tingling sensation or fullness, some may even experience a slight discomfort, while others may feel nothing at all.

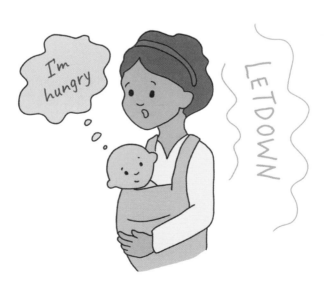

Breastmilk:
supply and demand

A breastfeeding mother and baby have an incredible relationship. Babies are perfect calorie regulators and will drink what they need – and a mother's body will (most of the time) respond perfectly to meet her baby's needs.

When a breastfeeding mother's hormones, breast tissue, nerve pathways and key nutrients are combined with effective milk removal and breast stimulation, **the result is direct milk production.**

Having the correct balance of these interactions ensures full production can be reached and sustained for as long as your baby demands.

The first weeks with your baby are vital for establishing a good long-term breastmilk supply.

The more frequently your baby breastfeeds, the more milk you'll make, through a process of supply and demand. Each time milk is removed from your breasts, either by your baby feeding or by you expressing, your body is signalled to rapidly refill the breasts in readiness for your baby's next feed.

Cluster feeding

Cluster feeding is when your baby's feeds are very frequent or 'clustered' together. During these periods, your baby seems to feed continuously over several hours, often in the evening or the early hours of the morning, and may not settle to sleep easily. This can be normal in the first four weeks of life (and beyond), as your baby intentionally increases your supply to meet their calorie needs. It can also be associated with low supply or sometimes comfort feeding, masking the true cause of unsettled behaviour.

If cluster feeding is happening regularly and your baby is frequently unsettled, it's worthwhile investigating further with your maternal health nurse, GP, lactation consultant or paediatrician.

> **After 4–6 weeks your milk is mature, and your production should be aligned with your baby's needs.**

- Your breasts will start to feel softer between feeds.

- For the next few months, your baby will take a similar volume of breastmilk each day, with occasional growth spurts and increased appetite causing temporary increases in volume.

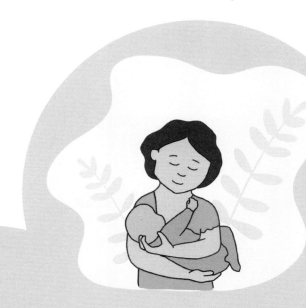

Below is a guide to how much breastmilk your baby will drink from birth up until six months. Keep in mind these are average amounts that vary considerably throughout the day and night. Age, size and feed frequency must also be taken into consideration.

AGE	AMOUNT PER FEED
First 24 hours	2–10 mL
Day 2	5–15 mL
Day 3	15–30 mL
Days 4–7	30–45 mL
1–2 weeks	45–60 mL
2–4 weeks	60–90 mL
1–6 months	60–120 mL

One way to know if your baby is receiving an adequate supply of breastmilk is via their nappies. By day 4–5, you should have at least five heavily wet nappies in 24 hours (light coloured urine). Healthcare professionals will look at this – in combination with baby's weight changes, examination findings, jaundice levels and feed frequency – to determine whether the supply is sufficient.

If you feel you have low supply, please discuss this with your health nurse, lactation consultant or local doctor.

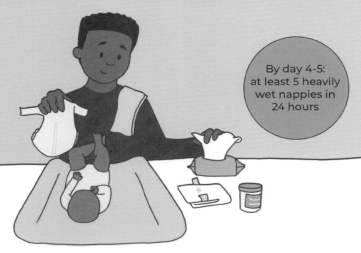

By day 4-5: at least 5 heavily wet nappies in 24 hours

You could also try these tips to build up supply:

- Offer both breasts at each feed. Return your baby to the first breast if baby is still hungry.

- Try switch feeding – five minutes at each breast, twice or more. This increases the number of 'letdowns' you have. Only do this if supply is low, otherwise you risk moving baby when there is still hindmilk to remove. This can cause lactose overload – see more on page 91.

See pg. 91

- Ensure your baby is correctly attached, as the breast will be drained more effectively.

- Express milk after feeds.

- Ensure you are eating well and drinking enough water. Your body will produce more milk when you look after yourself properly.

- Rest and relax as much as you can, especially during a feed.

- Breast compression or massage prior to and during a feed trigger ongoing letdowns, assisting your baby to remove the milk more efficiently.

- Enjoy as much skin-to-skin contact with your baby as possible. This is great for both breastmilk supply and bonding.

- Increase your intake of galactagogues (foods, herbs or medications that increase milk supply), such as wholegrains (especially oats), dark leafy greens, fennel, chickpeas, nuts (especially almonds), seeds and proteins.

Remember, though: not every mother is destined to exclusively breastfeed a baby; some not even for the first week. If you've tried these techniques and supply or attachment concerns remain, I urge you to speak to a lactation consultant, and also to consider that mix-feeding or exclusive bottle-feeding may be a more suitable option for you. Remember, if it feels right, then it is the right option for you.

Positioning
and attachment

Positioning and attachment are the prerequisites for successful breastfeeding. Breastfeeding a baby is often portrayed as a natural process after birth, but for many mothers it does not come naturally, and may require lots of patience and learning. This is perfectly natural, and does not reflect on your ability as a mother or parent!

Positioning

If a baby is positioned well at the breast, they will have the best chance of achieving an optimal latch, resulting in good milk transfer and a healthy milk supply.

There is no single right way to position your baby at the breast. The keys are:

a) for it to feel comfortable for both mother and baby

b) for there to be evidence of efficient colostrum/milk transfer e.g. deep, nutritive sucking (not using the nipple as a dummy) with regular swallowing, and breasts feeling softer after a feed.

Below are some examples of different positions you can try.

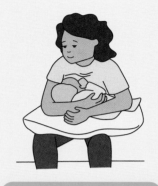

1. The cradle position

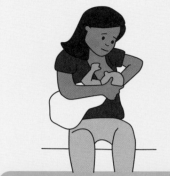

2. The cross-cradle position

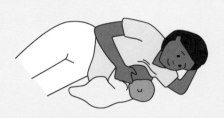

3. The side-lying position

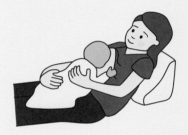

4. The laid-back position

If you are having difficulty getting your baby to latch at the breast, the laid-back position may be a good option. This position allows the baby to use their natural instincts to seek and attach to the breast without feeling pressure or force. It's also effective for slowing down the milk flow at the start of a feed if the letdowns are too fast.

Once a comfortable position has been established and the baby's chest and tummy are touching the mother's chest and tummy, it's time to attach to the breast.

Breast attachment

Correct attachment to the breast is often referred to as a 'good latch' and it's what will set you up for breastfeeding success. Some gentle support may be required initially to assist with correct attachment, but it won't take long for the baby to work out how to latch and suck properly.

Calmness while you find your confidence is the key. Remember, you and your baby are both learning together.

Tips for setting up the optimal environment to feed in:

Tip 1:
If the room is chaotic or you don't feel comfortable with people around, ask others to leave.

Tip 2:
Put on some calm music.

Tip 3:
Make sure you're wearing comfortable clothes:
- you don't want to be too hot or too cold
- ensure tops and bras are comfortable for breastfeeding – everyone is different.

Tip 4:
Have your drink bottle ready before you sit down.

Tip 5:
Turn off all other distractions, if you choose to.

Tip 6:
As you're learning, midwives will often physically help you (sometimes it's easier to show rather than tell). Be ready and open to this, as it can be very helpful. If you're not comfortable for whatever reason, speak up early.

Tip 7:
Watch for hunger signs and be conscious of the baby becoming overtired. It's very hard to effectively latch and feed a distraught newborn.

The five steps to breastfeeding

Step 1: Find a comfortable position first

- As discussed, there is no 'right way' to breastfeed, but you can start by sitting upright, with your back well supported.
- Soft couches or rocking chairs aren't ideal early on.
- If your baby is heavy or you've got a long torso, you can use a pillow to support your baby.

Step 2: Hold your baby close to your body

- Remember, if you're having to move your breast to reach your baby, you're not in the right position.
- Take care not to raise your baby higher than the natural fall of your breasts.

Step 3: Hold your baby behind their back and shoulders

- Your baby should be on their side with their chest touching your chest.
- Avoid placing your fingers on the back of the baby's head. This will interfere with the baby's ability to extend its neck and tilt its head back, which is crucial for effective suck/swallow and milk removal. Imagine someone pressing their finger on the back of your head while you're trying to have a drink.

Step 4: Bring your baby's nose just above your nipple

- Gently brush your nipple from your baby's nose to their lips. This will encourage your baby to open their mouth wide.

Step 5: When your baby's mouth is wide open, quickly bring your baby to your breast.

- Direct your nipple at the roof of your baby's mouth.
- Your baby will close their mouth over your breast, 'latch' and start sucking.

Tips on attachment

If your breasts are engorged or just very full, attachment can be hard.

Tip 1:
Try to express a small amount of milk to help soften the area around the areola.

Tip 2:
Shape your breast like a 'hamburger'

- You can do this by placing a thumb on the top of the breast with your fingers going under the breast, coming up on the inner side of the breast.
- A gentle squeeze of your hand will shape the breast and help your baby attach easier.
- This technique is likened to the way we squeeze a hamburger bun before we take a bite. It helps us get a bigger mouthful which is just what we want a baby to do.
- Continue to maintain the gentle squeeze until the baby has latched and is sucking effectively.
- Slowly let go of the breast once you feel confident the baby is breastfeeding well.

Think hamburger, not taco, as you position the breast into the baby's mouth to attach.

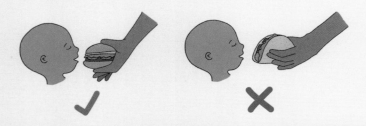

Signs that your baby is correctly attached:

- Breastfeeding feels comfortable, not painful.
- Your nipples stay in good condition and don't show any signs of damage or cracking.
- Your baby is sucking deeply and regularly, and you can see or hear baby swallowing. This is one of the best sounds in the world!
- Your baby's chin is pressed into your breast, and their nose is clear or just touching your breast.
- Your baby takes the whole nipple and a large amount of the areola into their mouth.
- Your baby's bottom lip is turned out over your breast (not sucked in), and their top lip is turned out or sitting softly on your breast.
- Your baby is draining your breast properly, so that it feels softer after a feed.

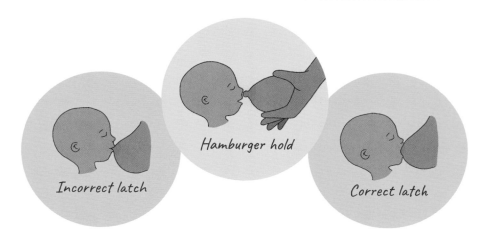

Incorrect latch

Hamburger hold

Correct latch

If you're in pain: Pain, particularly in the first few seconds after your baby attaches, usually means something is wrong. Break the suction by inserting your little finger into the corner of your baby's mouth, between the gums. Gently take your baby off the breast and try again.

Damaged nipples: Don't suffer through any pain when breastfeeding, as any nipple damage can impact your ability to feed. Don't push yourself until you break. If your nipples are damaged, you may need to rest them until they feel more comfortable. You have the option to express and feed your baby breastmilk via syringe, spoon, cup or bottle while your nipples heal.

Nipple shields are another option, and enable you to continue breastfeeding while giving your nipples time to heal. There are also protective silver healing covers and lanolin-based creams you can use to help speed up recovery.

Being empowered when breastfeeding: If you want to double-check your position and your baby's attachment, or if you have any other breastfeeding concerns, I urge you to contact a lactation consultant early. Other professionals such as your midwife, child and family health nurse, or breastfeeding association counsellor may also be able to assist. Don't wait – establishing milk supply and pain-free feeding in the first days will set you up for long-term success.

Breast fullness and engorgement

Breast fullness or engorgement is likely to occur anytime from 24 hours post-birth, when an increase in milk, blood and lymphatic fluid causes heavy, swollen breasts that can make attachment difficult.

While this can be a normal part of the process of breastfeeding, it can lead to:

1. a sudden reduction in milk supply
2. mastitis, if not attended to quickly. See pages 98–99 for more on mastitis.

A drainage technique called reverse pressure softening can soften the tissue at the base of the nipple, helping your baby gain a deeper latch and improving the transfer of milk from breast to baby. A small amount of milk is expressed off, either using a pump or by hand, to soften the areola, making it easier for the baby to attach.

If your baby is unable to remove the milk effectively, a pump may be required until your baby is ready and able to feed from the breast. Sometimes women get relief from a single pump, removing all the milk from their breasts just once. This softens the breasts, making them more comfortable, and makes it easier for your baby to attach and suck.

Prevention:

- Ensure correct position/attachment during feeds.
- Drain breast fully before switching sides.
- Unrestricted breastfeeding (or expressing) 8–12 times in 24 hours.
- Avoid skipping night feeds.

Engorgement management:

- Avoid hot showers on breast tissue, as this can overstimulate and increase swelling.
- Use a warm compress on the breast prior to breastfeeding to stimulate the letdown reflex.
- Express, either by hand or using a pump, to remove a small amount of milk prior to breastfeeding, or use the reverse pressure softening technique to soften the tissue around the base of the nipple before attaching the baby to the breast.
- If the baby only breastfeeds on one side and the other breast is uncomfortable, express enough milk out of the other side to soften the breast, for comfort only.
- Use cool packs on the breast after a feed to help reduce swelling and discomfort.
- Talk to your doctor about the use of anti-inflammatories or pain relief should the swelling and discomfort continue.
- Avoid skipping night feeds.

Inverted, flat and short nipples

A large percentage of women have nipples that are inverted, flat or short, and this can make breastfeeding difficult.

If this affects you, good and early support can help your baby latch successfully without causing any damage to the nipple or breast tissue.

If your baby is unable to latch, it is important not to push them to breastfeed, as this can lead to a frustrated and angry baby who may start to show signs of breast refusal. It is far better to keep your baby calm and relaxed by giving some milk to satisfy their initial hunger, then bring them back to your chest for skin-to-skin contact and cuddles.

Your key focus at this point is to establish a good milk supply as quickly as possible so that you can:

1. have milk to give your baby

2. return your baby to the breast as soon as possible, once the milk volume has increased. Your baby will suck much better once the milk is flowing.

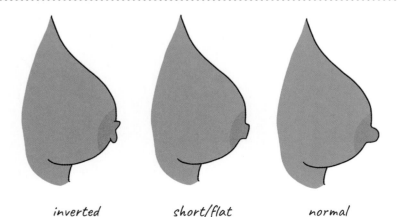

inverted   short/flat   normal

Nipple shields

- You may find that initially, you need to use a nipple shield when returning your baby to the breast, until your baby feels comfortable and trusts that the breast will deliver the milk volume needed.

- Check in with a lactation consultant or maternal nurse for guidance on correct sizing and usage.

- It's possible, once your baby is breastfeeding well, that you will no longer need the nipple shield. This will depend on the degree of your nipple inversion or damage.

- If you attempt to remove the shield, make sure you remove it after the baby has had enough milk to feel relaxed and content, but still wants to continue feeding. If the shield is removed too soon and your baby is unable to latch onto the nipple, they may protest and become angry.

- Some mums may only need to use the shield to initially draw out the nipple.

- If you use a nipple shield, it is important that you can see and hear the milk transfer (as your baby swallows milk). You will see milk in the shield, your breasts will soften as the feed progresses and your baby will start to slow down, with longer pauses between sucking.

- To ensure the breast is well drained and the baby gets as much of the rich, creamy milk as possible, use gentle hand massage and compression. This will help stimulate removal of the remaining milk and ensure your baby is full and content.

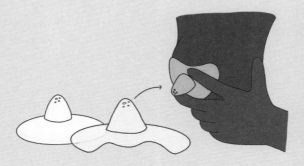

Maternal nutrition and hydration

When you're breastfeeding, your body needs extra nutrients. That's because your body is working harder to make breastmilk that is full of nutrients for your baby.

A note on hydration:

While hydration is the key, excess water is not required to increase the supply of breastmilk.

In fact, too much water can be detrimental to breastmilk supply and can even cause swollen/engorged breasts. A mother should drink to quench thirst. If breastfeeding makes you feel thirsty then you should drink, but not excessive amounts of water in the belief that it will make more milk. This is an old wives' tale.

What to eat when breastfeeding

Producing breastmilk requires energy.

Some women find they need to increase their normal diet by up to 50 per cent, or an extra 400–500 calories per day, to make enough milk to meet their baby's needs. Extra body fat gained during pregnancy is one way of providing mothers with the necessary calories needed to produce milk.

For mothers keen to reduce weight after delivery, it's important to consider a gradual return to pre-birth weight. Any sudden weight loss can result in a dramatic decrease in milk production due to the sudden loss of body fat.

The recommended daily intake for breastfeeding mothers is:

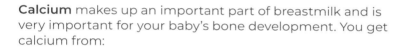

- ☑ vegetables – 7½ serves a day
- ☑ fruit – 2 serves a day
- ☑ grain foods – 9 serves a day
- ☑ protein – 2½ serves a day
- ☑ dairy or calcium-enriched products – 2½ serves a day.

If you're eating a healthy and varied diet, you will get enough of most nutrients, but there are a few to be specifically aware of.

Calcium makes up an important part of breastmilk and is very important for your baby's bone development. You get calcium from:

- dairy products like milk, cheese and yoghurt (be aware of possible cow milk intolerance in babies)
- calcium-enriched products, like some brands of soy milk
- fish with edible bones, like sardines and salmon
- tofu
- green leafy vegetables like kale and bok choy
- white beans, figs, sesame seeds, almonds, broccoli and seaweed.

Note: A breastfeeding mother's body will always prioritise the nutritional needs of the baby. This means that any calcium will be directed to the baby first, which emphasises the importance of maintaining the mother's own calcium levels while breastfeeding.

Zinc is a crucial ingredient in our immune system. It can be found in red meat, poultry, beans, nuts, oats, seeds and seafood.

Omega 3 fatty acids occur naturally in flaxseeds, chia seeds, salmon, walnuts, tofu, oysters, canola oil, brussels sprouts and avocados.

Iodine helps with the brain and nervous system development. You get iodine from dairy products, seafood, iodised salt, potatoes, cheese, cranberries, tuna, shellfish and dried prunes. Iodine deficiency in breastfeeding mothers can be a risk for babies. When you're breastfeeding, it's recommended that you take an iodine supplement of 150 micrograms (µg) per day. If you have any pre-existing thyroid problems, check with your doctor before taking a supplement.

Vitamin B12 is very important for your baby's blood and developing nervous system. You get vitamin B12 from meat, fish (especially shellfish and tuna), eggs, milk, yoghurt, brewer's yeast and fortified breakfast cereals. Those on vegetarian/vegan diets or taking antibiotics or anti-inflammatories may have reduced vitamin B12 levels.

Vitamin D helps your baby absorb calcium, which they will need for bone growth and development. Your body makes most of the vitamin D you need from exposure to sunlight. There are also small amounts of vitamin D in oily fish, fish oil supplements, egg yolks, mushrooms, milk, ricotta cheese and butter. You might be at risk of vitamin D deficiency if you're dark-skinned, keep all of your skin covered or rarely go outdoors. If you're deficient, you and your baby might need to take a vitamin D supplement.

Iron helps the body make haemoglobin, the major part of red blood cells, helping us deliver oxygen around the body. When iron-deficient – or anaemic – you may experience lower energy levels. To increase your iron, eat more brown rice, soybeans, oysters, chicken, beef, turkey, lentils, tofu, nuts, seeds and green leafy vegetables. To further maximise your iron absorption, when eating these foods, add some vitamin C (from citrus fruits) and be sure to avoid excess dairy, as this reduces iron absorption.

Fluid intake is crucial, and never more so than when breastfeeding. Most mothers will attest to insatiable thirst during the breastfeeding period – this is not surprising, given the water content of breastmilk! The recommended 2 litres per day is a good starting point, but drink more if you remain thirsty. Be careful not to drink excessive amounts; excessive water intake does not result in more milk production and can worsen oedema (swelling). Avoid soft drinks, fruit juices, flavoured milk, flavoured water, sports drinks and energy drinks.

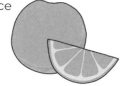

Vegan and vegetarian mothers may experience lower milk supply or fatigue due to reduced B12 intake. Calcium, protein and iron levels may also be reduced. To help the body absorb iron, add foods high in vitamin C such as citrus fruits. For protein, consider plant sources, such as soy products and meat substitutes, legumes, lentils, nuts, seeds and whole grains. For calcium, include dairy products (unless vegan), dark green vegetables, calcium-enriched and fortified products, such as juices, cereals, soy milk, soy yoghurt and tofu. There is no need to eat against your beliefs, but have your nutrient levels checked and supplement these if any are low. This is not only important for your baby, it's also crucial for you and your general health.

What not to eat when breastfeeding

Global breastfeeding associations recommend that no particular foods be excluded from a breastfeeding mother's diet, unless advised by a doctor. Research confirms that excluding particular allergenic foods from the breastfeeding mother's diet does not reduce the likelihood of her child developing allergies.

With any sensible diet ...

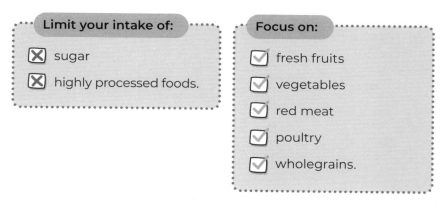

Limit your intake of:
- [X] sugar
- [X] highly processed foods.

Focus on:
- [✓] fresh fruits
- [✓] vegetables
- [✓] red meat
- [✓] poultry
- [✓] wholegrains.

These will give you the sustained energy needed for managing a newborn and breastfeeding a baby.

Your baby is exposed to everything you eat.

Some babies are sensitive to certain foods, like milk, garlic or broccoli, whereas others can tolerate their mother eating any and every food type. If you notice a change in your baby's behaviour, bowel actions or skin in the days following a change in your diet, consider that they may be sensitive to something you ate.

If you're breastfeeding, be aware of your diet, particularly if you're consuming a lot of:

cow's milk

roughage

fermented products

legumes

cured meats

These could upset your baby. Remember, food that makes you gassy, will make your baby gassy, too.

Caffeine and breastmilk

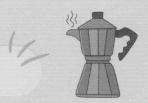

Please note: This section is not intended to stop your morning coffee ritual

I hate focusing on this too much, as breastfeeding is one of the toughest jobs out there – and mums need their coffee more than anyone!

BUT if you have an unsettled baby who is struggling with sleep, it's important to understand the impact of caffeine on breastmilk.

Newborn babies can be sensitive to caffeine.

Your newborn baby will take a significant amount of time to process the caffeine that comes through your breastmilk – which can remain in your system for up to 50 hours.

The effects caffeine can have on babies include:

- jitteriness
- more unsettled behaviour
- difficulty sleeping
- increased colicky behaviour
- general unhappiness.

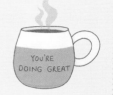

YOU'RE
DOING GREAT

Be aware that caffeine isn't just in coffee. It's also found in:

- tea
- chocolate
- cola
- energy drinks.

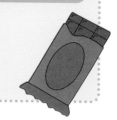

How much caffeine is transferred to my baby?

The amount of caffeine that transfers into your breastmilk is about 1 per cent of what is consumed, and reaches a peak 60 minutes after consumption.

It is recommended not to consume more than 200 mg of caffeine per day.

Caffeine content in common drinks and food

Drink/Food	Caffeine level (mg)
Espresso coffee	145 mg/50 mL shot
Formulated caffeinated (energy) drinks	up to 80 mg/250 mL can
Instant coffee (1 teaspoon/cup)	60–80 mg/250 mL cup
Tea	10–50 mg/250 mL cup
Cola	up to 54 mg/375 mL cup
Milk chocolate	20 mg/100 g bar
Dark chocolate	up to 85 mg/100g bar

Alcohol and breastmilk

The amount of alcohol in your blood is the same as the amount of alcohol in your breastmilk.

It is generally safe to enjoy an alcoholic drink, but there are a few factors to take into consideration, including:

- your weight
- your food intake
- alcohol strength
- volume consumed
- timing of breastfeeds.

Alcohol will appear in your blood 30–60 minutes after you begin drinking, so if you do wish to enjoy an alcoholic drink, it is safest to do so immediately after a feed.

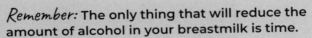

Remember: **The only thing that will reduce the amount of alcohol in your breastmilk is time.**

If you plan to have a drink, the Australian Breastfeeding Association (ABA) has a great app, Feed Safe, which will time how long you need to wait before breastfeeding after drinking.

Lactose overload – the foremilk and hindmilk imbalance

Your breastmilk is made up of a combination of both foremilk and hindmilk.

Foremilk is the milk your baby has at the beginning of the feed. It is a low-fat, high lactose (sugar) milk that flows out quickly from the breast during the first few letdowns. It provides immediate satisfaction and often allows a hungry baby to then settle in for a longer feed and reach the hindmilk.

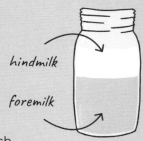

Hindmilk is the remaining milk, which is rich, creamy and high in fat. Hindmilk is great for helping your baby gain weight and feel a sense of fullness. Due to its high fat content, it sometimes attaches to the milk cell walls, making it hard for your letdowns to eject it out of the breast. If this happens, a light hand massage and gentle shake of the breast while leaning forward will mix up the milk and make it easier for your baby to remove all the breastmilk.

The difference between foremilk and hindmilk is more dynamic and nuanced than two distinct milk types, but thinking about it in this way can help identify lactose overload.

Lactose overload can occur if your baby is consuming too much foremilk and not enough hindmilk.

> *Note:* These measures are usually only temporary until your breasts recalibrate to meet your baby's needs. As your baby grows bigger and stronger, they will be able to remove the hindmilk more effectively from your breasts.

Problems that can occur from not getting enough hindmilk:

- You may find your baby fills up on the foremilk and does not stay attached long enough to also remove the hindmilk.
- Not removing the hindmilk means your baby will feed more frequently, having foremilk-only feeds. As foremilk contains lactose (regardless of a mother's diet), this can result in lactose overload.
- Baby's behaviour becomes more irritable and unsettled, with gas and wind causing your baby pain.
- Baby's poo may become greener in colour and loose or 'frothy' in consistency. This can lead to painful nappy rash (dermatitis).

An imbalance can be caused by:

- Moving your baby from one breast to the other too quickly, before your baby has had the chance to drain the breast.

Tips to help your baby access more hindmilk:

- Try not to move your baby to the other breast too quickly when you know there is more milk in your breast.
- If your baby is sleepy at the breast, use gentle hand massage and compression of the breast during and towards the end of the feed. This will help your breast eject the remaining hindmilk more efficiently.
- If your baby continues to be sleepy you may need to use a pump to remove the remaining hindmilk to bottle-feed to them later. This will help maintain your supply and avoid complications such as engorgement and mastitis.

Remember: This section isn't meant to cause unnecessary worry about timed feedings in the first 4 weeks. Overall, most babies get what they need over a 24-hour period. It's just a reminder not to rush a feed, or move from one breast to the other too quickly, and to keep an eye out for signs of lactose overload in nappies.

Other complications

Babies that are premature, small for gestational age, jaundiced or have severe tongue-tie are at greater risk of lactose overload due to their lack of strength, tone and ability to sustain a breastfeed long enough to drain the breast.

These babies:

- are likely to breastfeed for short periods of time and shouldn't be pushed to feed at the breast any longer than physically capable.
- should be given the rich, creamy hindmilk during each feed to ensure they continue to gain weight and thrive. How you give this to your baby is up to you.

You may find:

- a feeding supplement device at the breast, such as a supply line, works well, as this keeps the baby attached to the breast and avoids possible breast refusal. With a supply line it becomes easier for a baby to feed as they don't have to work as hard, so it can be great for babies who tire easily at the breast. These sorts of supplementary nursing systems are introduced by lactation consultants.
- your baby is simply too tired and needs to be fed in the quickest and easiest way possible to avoid loss of energy and weight. This may mean using a bottle until your baby is strong enough to manage a full breastfeed without fatiguing.

Breastmilk and formula

When talking about newborns and babies, there is no topic that ignites more emotion-charged debate and angst than that of breastmilk versus formula.

There's no getting around it: exclusive breastfeeding is definitely better for the baby. No arguments there. But this is not always possible – and what's best for the baby may not necessarily be best for the mother.

> What sometimes gets lost in this debate is this: **protecting the physical and mental wellbeing of mothers is key**.

As a paediatrician, my singular focus is the wellbeing of the baby, but the most effective tool I have as a doctor is the baby's mother. That's why so much of what I do revolves around:

- protecting the mother
- maximising her wellbeing
- cultivating a strong, connected mother–baby relationship.

As a member of the Australian Breastfeeding Association for Health Professionals, I work closely with lactation consultants every single day – as well as through my sleep programs and this book – to promote breastfeeding, work on increasing supply and troubleshoot whenever possible.

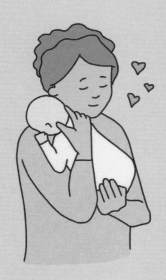

I am pro-breastfeeding, but not at the cost of the wellbeing of the mother and the mother–baby relationship.

> **A breastfeeding mother's general health and wellbeing can be compromised by:**
>
> - the stress and sleep deprivation associated with more frequent night feeds
> - some pro-lactation medications
> - guilt
> - fear
> - perceived judgement
> - the pressure to exclusively breastfeed.
>
> **Remember rule #1: there is no room for judgement.**

Put your own oxygen mask on first.

On day one of medical school, we are taught DRSABC. The D stands for danger – we are always taught to think of our own safety first, before addressing the wellbeing of others.

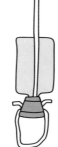

This is just like putting on your own oxygen mask first before helping your child, as in in-flight safety demonstrations. If we are injured or incapacitated, we are of no use to anyone.

The same thing applies to mothers.

Call it *survival strategy* if you like. If a mother protects her own wellbeing through good nutrition, rest and emotional support, she will be more likely to meet the needs of her baby.

Breastfeeding is great, but let's look at the data.

When it works well, exclusive breastfeeding is brilliant. It's efficient, it's healthy for mother and baby, it's portable, sterile – it's absolutely magical. And it's like forced mindfulness, requiring patience, cuddling and unhurried emotional connections during both day and night.

When it works, it's beautiful, and without question the best food source for babies. Centuries of research have left no doubt about the benefits of breastfeeding for babies and mothers.

For babies, these benefits include:

- decreased infection rates
- lower risk of diabetes, leukaemia and obesity.

For mothers, these benefits include:

- a lower risk of breast and ovarian cancer
- lower rates of obesity.

What's not often talked about is the *degree* of the benefit of exclusive breastfeeding. If a mother is told that breastfeeding will reduce her baby's risk of leukaemia by 15 per cent – as some studies demonstrate – she will do everything she can to continue breastfeeding in order to protect her child.

That's natural – and beautiful.

But let's look at what those numbers really mean. Let's get some perspective here. Childhood leukaemia – as an example – is not common. It occurs in roughly four in 100,000 children. A 15 per cent reduction brings that frequency down from four to 3.4 in 100,000 children. So while the percentage reduction sounds large, the actual numbers are tiny.

This statistic needs to be weighed up against all the other factors that relate to the health of the mother, and the mother–baby relationship.

The pressure to exclusively breastfeed.

All too often, I see women trying to adjust their bodies to fit a social construct of 'the perfect mother'. But exclusive breastfeeding isn't always possible, and your baby may need to be fed in a different way. That's okay.

No matter which way you choose to feed your baby, be it with breastmilk, breastmilk and formula (mixed), donor milk or formula, your baby will be fine. They will continue to receive the same love and connection you have always shared, regardless of the way the milk is delivered.

Adding formula top-ups does NOT undo the benefits of breastmilk and breastfeeding. In my practice, I have found that mothers who shift to mixed feeding (when supply wanes) actually end up breastfeeding for longer, compared with those who persist with exclusive breastfeeding.

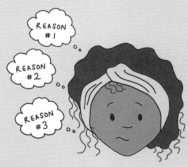

A depressed, exhausted or anxious mother isn't able to provide the nurturing that a baby so desperately needs. If that mother's state is worsened by an overwhelming pressure to exclusively breastfeed, it's just not worthwhile.

Not all women were born with the ability to exclusively breastfeed a child. This has always been the case. A woman's ability to breastfeed is influenced by any number of factors, such as:

- the birth experience
- hormone changes
- supply issues
- inverted or flat nipples
- pain
- sleep deprivation
- maternal mental health
- previous abuse or trauma
- the baby's oral anatomy, gestation and size.

In tribal areas, some women were hunters, some were teachers and some were wet nurses. The women who produced copious volumes of milk and had perfectly shaped nipples were tasked with feeding all the babies of the tribe. Everybody had a way of contributing, and no woman was judged for going out hunting while another mother took care of the breastfeeding.

In fact, in the eighteenth and nineteenth centuries, wet nursing became a potential career! Unfortunately, aristocracy regarded breastfeeding as a lower-class practice, so it was often outsourced.

Today, however, we don't live in tribes. We know it takes a *village* to raise a child, but here we are, living mostly segregated, isolated lives in individual homes.

And sadly, women who aren't able to exclusively breastfeed their children can be overcome by guilt and anxiety, prompting them to pursue excessive measures in their determination to exclusively breastfeed – measures that ignore the individual circumstances of the mother.

Signs that exclusive breastfeeding may not be working or not be right for you:

- Your baby might not seem satisfied after a feed.
- They might not be urinating much.
- They might not be gaining adequate weight.
- They might be feeding too frequently.

Separately, you might be experiencing:

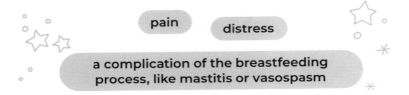

pain

distress

a complication of the breastfeeding process, like mastitis or vasospasm

Mastitis

Mastitis is an inflammatory complication of breastfeeding that occurs when the breast becomes inflamed because of blocked milk ducts and/or damaged nipples.

Breast tenderness, redness and painful lumps, together with flu-like symptoms such as fever, shivers and body aches, are all common symptoms. Up to one in five mothers experience mastitis, sometimes multiple times. Prevention and early intervention/treatment are essential – it presents and progresses incredibly quickly.

Prevention:

- Drain the breast often, around 8–12 times in 24 hours (use a pump if baby is not able to effectively remove the milk).
- Avoid skipping the night feed or delaying breastfeeds in the first weeks.
- Offer both breasts if possible. If the baby is not able to remove any milk from the second breast, use a pump to remove enough milk for comfort, then offer the second breast first at the next feed.
- Ensure the baby is positioned and latched correctly.
- Massage the breast during feeding, as this helps release more milk for your baby. A great time to do this is when you notice your baby is not sucking, or is becoming sleepy at the breast. You will notice your baby starts to suck and swallow as the letdown occurs.
- Wear a supportive bra – always make sure these are fitted correctly and not too firm or tight, as that can be a contributing factor to mastitis.

Treatment:

- Rest between feeds.
- Consider analgesia (pain relief).
- Use warm compresses for a few minutes before breastfeeding to help you relax and to stimulate letdown.
- Use cool packs intermittently after and between breastfeeds to help soothe painful breasts and reduce inflammation.
- If unresolved after 24 hours and you are feeling unwell or your breasts are red, tender and becoming lumpy, contact your doctor, as you may need antibiotics.
- Keep feeding your baby from the breast if possible, as this is the best way to keep draining the milk and prevent blocked ducts.
- Ultrasound therapy can be effective – usually only one or two treatments are needed. This can reduce inflammation, unblock ducts and help clear infection.

Vasospasm

Nipple vasospasm is what happens when the blood vessels supplying the nipple go into spasm and reduce the blood flow to the nipple. This affects the flow of milk from the nipple. It is common to feel an intense throbbing or burning pain if this happens, particularly if the weather is cold.

Some women are more likely to have nipple vasospasm, particularly those who have pre-existing poor circulation (like cold hands and feet). Women who are below average weight for their height are also at greater risk. Cigarette smoking can make vasospasm worse, because nicotine constricts the blood vessels.

You can manage the effects of nipple vasospasm by reducing your exposure to the air or cold or wearing warmer layers. This will help your blood vessels to stay dilated and avoid becoming restricted.

> If you think you might be suffering from one of these breastfeeding conditions – speak to a lactation consultant or doctor about treatment and simple measures that might help improve the process.

Alternative options

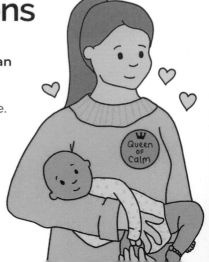

When breastfeeding isn't going to plan it is important that the mother feels supported, reassured and not judged. Stress and pressure do not help anyone.

Remember – babies drink much more than milk. They drink your warmth, your love, your connectedness.

But they also drink your anxiety, your worry, your stress, your guilt and your fear.

In my practice, when you remove that pressure to exclusively breastfeed if things aren't going according to plan, I have found that breastfeeding actually continues for much longer. It's as if a mother is given 'emotional permission' to mix-feed her baby, which prolongs the benefits to both mother and child.

Formula arrived in the mid-nineteenth century, devised by Henri Nestlé in 1867. That name should ring a bell – Henri invented formula just prior to establishing his partnership with chocolatier Daniel Peter, with whom he created Nestlé chocolate! As a result, mothers who aren't exclusively breastfeeding have the choice between feeding their baby expressed milk, donor milk and formula, or a combination of all of these.

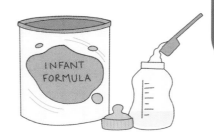

Donor milk is expressed breastmilk that is donated via formal 'milk banks' or informally through private channels. Formal banks have screening processes in place to ensure donor mothers are healthy and milk is usually pasteurised to remove any viruses and bacteria from the stored milk.

If you're not having problems with breastfeeding, it's wise to avoid introducing formula until your breastmilk is properly established (around 4–6 weeks). However, if you need to introduce formula for the wellbeing of yourself or your baby, there are many options available to help protect your milk supply while you enjoy the benefits of mixed feeding.

Don't push yourself until you break. That benefits nobody, least of all your baby.

Supplementing your baby's intake with formula – to meet their requirements – is perfectly fine. Always.

A final note to all mothers:

If you are a mother who loves her child, who protects her child, who nurtures her child – you are perfect. If you can't exclusively breastfeed, or if you don't want to, you are no less of a mother and should never be made to feel that way.

Mothers need reassurance and support – not judgement.

Make the decision that feels right for you and your growing family. As a paediatrician, I know how important it is to never pressure you or make you feel guilty or ashamed when exclusive breastfeeding is not possible or not your personal choice.

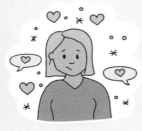

Remember, the many benefits of breastfeeding are not undone by the addition of formula. In fact, more potential benefits arise when a bottle is introduced, such as enabling dads to get in on the feeding action. This provides enormous support for mums and is shown to dramatically reduce the incidence of paternal postnatal depression, unlocking a vital source of oxytocin in dads – the hormone that drives protective instincts.

So no matter which way you choose to feed your baby, feel proud that you are giving them the best start in life by providing all the love, nutrition and security they require.

And remember, always – nourish yourself first. Then feed your baby.

Breast and bottle

After giving birth, circumstances sometimes require a baby to be fed with a bottle.

The baby may have been premature, making it difficult to feed at the breast, or the mother's nipples may be highly sensitive, damaged or shaped in a way that makes it difficult for her baby to latch properly.

Delayed lactation is another reason many women introduce bottles in the early days.

Whether you choose to breastfeed or bottle-feed (or a combination of both), the decision is a personal one.

Consideration is always given to meeting a baby's nutritional needs and implementing ongoing feeding plans that support your wishes and capabilities moving forward.

	PROS	CONS
Breastfeeding	· Ready when your baby is ready. No preparation required. · Has all the nutrients baby needs · Boosts baby's immune system · Protects fragile gut systems · Reduces risk of SIDS · Breastmilk is free	· Discomfort or pain, and challenges in some cases, especially early on · Supply issues · Frequent feeding · Only the breastfeeding parent can do it
Bottle (breastmilk and/or formula)	· Can feed your baby breastmilk and formula · Easy for compromised babies still developing sucking and strength · Dad + family + caretaker can feed baby · Easy to see how much milk baby is drinking	· Bottle refusal · Breast refusal · Overfeeding · Cleaning and sterilising · Lacks some nutrients (formula) · Can be inconvenient during night feeds or when out of the home · Formula is more expensive than breastmilk

Milk intolerances

I regularly hear mothers express concern that their baby is allergic to something in their breastmilk.

It is extremely important to highlight the difference between **allergy** and **intolerance**.

Babies can't be allergic to their mother's milk.

It is possible, however, for the baby to be intolerant to something the breastfeeding mother has consumed in their own diet and passed on to the baby via the milk.

An intolerance means that more exposure results in more symptoms. This is unlike allergy, where even the smallest exposure triggers a reaction.

Note: Intolerances are common in both bottle-fed and breastfed babies.

Common symptoms of intolerance include:

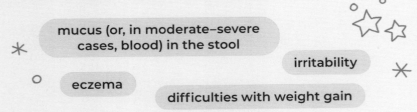

mucus (or, in moderate–severe cases, blood) in the stool

irritability

eczema

difficulties with weight gain

The most common foods babies can be intolerant to are:

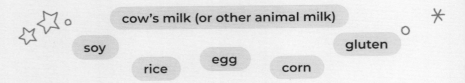

cow's milk (or other animal milk)

soy

gluten

rice

egg

corn

Mucus in poo

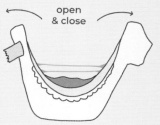

You can see mucus in poo by its shine.
If you hold the nappy together and pull
it apart you'll see strings, like power lines.
Mucus in the poo is a sign of inflammation.

What to do if you think your baby is intolerant to something

- If you're seeing a lot of mucusy poos, my first
  recommendation is to think about exclusion.
- If your baby is bottle fed, you may want to try a
  non-cow's-milk-based formula.
- If you're breastfeeding, you may want to decrease
  or avoid the consumption of cow's milk products.

Breastfeeding and exclusion diets

- It can take a while (2–3 days) for a food group to leave your
  system, and then another couple of days to see results in your
  baby. Don't expect things to change overnight – it can be a bit
  of a process.
- If limiting cow's milk doesn't help, try soy next. For the majority of
  babies this should solve the problem. If you're still seeing mucus
  and discomfort, follow the list at the base of page 104 in order.
- This shouldn't be militant – breastfeeding is one of the hardest
  jobs out there. If your baby has strong weight gain, is settled and
  is sleeping well, there's no reason to deprive yourself of essential
  food. Small amounts of mucus can be tolerated.
- Breastfeeding diets need to stay balanced. If you're removing
  food groups from your diet, talk to your GP about how to ensure
  you're getting all the nutrients you need. This is also important
  to help you keep up your milk supply.
- Once the poos have been normal for a while, you can slowly
  reintroduce the foods you excluded to your diet. If
  your baby stays happy and the poos stay normal,
  you'll know that you're back on track.
- Depending on severity, you can trial the foods again
  after about a month.

Some notes on intolerances/mucus in poo

- As discussed, while it is a sign of inflammation, mucus in the poo is not the end of the world. If your baby has strong weight gain, is settled and is sleeping well, there is no need to panic.
- If your baby is irritable, having trouble sleeping or if their weight gain is problematic, it may be something worth investigating further.

Remember: As always, this advice is general. If you are concerned about intolerances, discuss them with your baby's doctor.

Dairy allergy

Dairy allergy (including anaphylaxis) is not common and is very different to an intolerance.

If a baby is allergic to dairy, this won't be triggered by their mother's milk. If offering formula for the first time, start with a small volume to ensure there's no reaction before increasing to larger volumes.

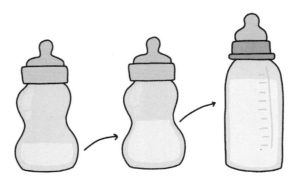

Growth charts and weight centiles

What is a baby or infant growth chart?

An infant growth chart helps you, your doctor, maternal nurses and other health professionals keep track of how your baby is growing.

Growth charts record changes in your baby's measurements, including their:

- length (height)
- weight
- head circumference

These measurements will be recorded on your baby's physical and/or digital records.

Your baby's growth is a good indicator of their overall health, nutrition and development.

What are centile charts?

Like us, babies come in all shapes and sizes. Centile charts work simply by comparing your baby's growth with other babies of the same age – the charts differ by gender (different charts exist for certain medical conditions too).

Baby centile and infant growth charts are usually calculated using the World Health Organization's growth standards.

You will see the percentile lines on the chart running parallel to each other.

The percentile lines include 5%, 10%, 25%, 50%, 75%, 90% and 95%.

Example 1:
If a child's weight is at the 50th percentile line, that means that out of 100 children of that age, 50 will be bigger than they are, and 50 smaller.

Example 2:
If a child's weight is in the 75th percentile, that means that your baby is bigger than 75 children and smaller than 25, compared with 100 children their own age.

Example 3:
A baby on the 5th percentile weighs less than 95% of other babies of that age.

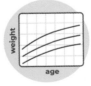

When it comes to measuring our babies on these curves, it's important to remember some babies will always be small, and others will always be large. You haven't mastered parenting if your baby is in the 90th percentile, and you're not a failure if your baby is in the 10th percentile! Where they sit is less important than their rate of growth.

Initial weight loss in newborns

When a baby is growing in utero, their mother is managing their body waste disposal, meaning the developing foetal kidneys have very little work to do. When the baby is born, the kidneys very slowly begin to turn on, and start filtering blood to excrete waste in the form of urine.

The amount of urine produced initially is so small and concentrated that when seen in the newborn nappy, it is often mistaken for blood. This urine (or urate crystals) quickly dissipates as feed volume increases and the kidneys rapidly improve their function.

By day 2–3 of life, the kidneys begin 'diuresing' – meaning that a large volume of body fluid is turned into urine and flushed out. This large fluid shift almost always results in an initial drop in weight, prior to baby beginning to gain weight.

Your baby will be weighed on day three. We generally tolerate a maximum drop of 10 per cent of birth weight before becoming concerned about milk adequacy.

Following the curve

All babies grow at different rates, and 'normal' growth varies.

The thing your health care professional will be looking for is that your baby continues to grow at a similar rate – this is often referred to as 'following the curve'.

But their growth won't always follow a smooth linear path on these curves, so be sure to put the growth charts and centiles into context. Babies and infants will often bounce up and down slightly on the growth charts, depending on feeding issues, illnesses etc.

Don't obsess about every movement on your baby's growth chart. When there is a persistent downward trend, this should always be investigated by a health professional.

Dropping centiles in the first months of life

I often encounter 2–3-month-olds referred for concerns regarding faltering weight. While weight reduction requires medical attention, a more common scenario arises where a baby's weight is increasing in a beautiful way, but their centiles are dropping.

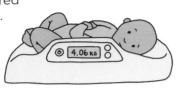

Now before we continue, there is a caveat: weight stagnation (or loss) in a baby, especially in the setting of poor feeding, development concerns, low tone or any other sign or symptom, needs full investigation.

But ... often a scenario emerges. A baby looks to be thriving and has a perfect examination, there's adequate milk supply, all investigations for growth failure come up normal with no major concerns from the parents – just a baby gaining weight but dropping from, say, the 80th centile to the 50th.

> This could be a **weight correction**, which is when a baby is born at a higher centile than they are genetically likely to remain at, so the loss in centiles is simply a 'correction' driven by genetics.

There are a few things we need to consider when discussing the possibility of a *weight correction*.

To fully understand this concept, let's go back to the womb. During gestation, the size of the baby is determined by many factors, including:

- the health of the placenta
- the umbilical cord
- the possibility of gestational diabetes
- gestation length
- maternal blood pressure.

Once the baby is born, assuming we're talking about a well baby, who is feeding and growing happily at home, with an adequate milk supply, their weight is determined more by their:

a) feeding patterns   b) genetics.

Take, for example, a baby born to two parents who themselves sit low on weight centiles, yet with a mother affected by gestational diabetes who delivers a baby on the 90th centile. This baby is highly unlikely to live on the 90th centile for life. If they were genetically predetermined to be closer to the 15th centile, for example, they will grow and thrive, but will steadily drop down the centiles (always growing in weight, but dropping in centiles) until they reach the 15th centile.

This commonly occurs in the first few months of life and can explain the drop in centiles, despite the presence of a perfectly happy, healthy baby.

It is crucial to remember that any drop in centiles needs to be monitored closely and the threshold for referral should remain low. But once more concerning problems have been comfortably excluded, we can rest assured that this baby is still thriving, while simply finding their place on the centiles chart.

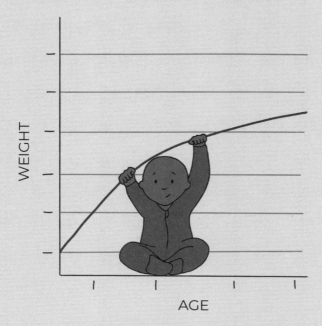

66

Welcome home!

While hospital can be exhausting, with lights
and noises and the regular monitoring of baby and
mother, there's the added benefit that someone brings
you meals, helps you with breastfeeding and keeps the
sheets clean. But getting home is another story.

99

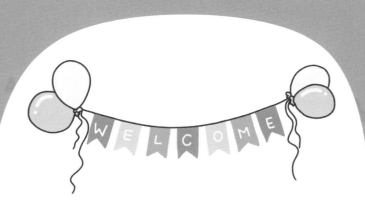

The first four weeks of *parenthood*

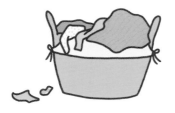

This is where your postpartum preparation, and encouragement of friends and family to give you 'doing gifts' for the first four weeks really comes in handy!

Before you keep reading this section, I want to reassure you that there's no better parent for your baby than you.

Walk in the door with your shoulders back. Take a big breath and know that not every day/hour/minute is going to be perfect – but you're empowered with the knowledge of what to expect and when you may need help. Never be afraid to ask for help if you need it.

You've got this!

Babies 'wake up' at 3–4 weeks

One thing that surprises most new parents is that babies can be incredibly oblivious to loud noises when they first arrive home.

You can take a newborn to a loud restaurant or rock concert, and they'll probably sleep soundly, despite the noise.

They'll also sleep in a central living area with full light and the bustle of a busy home.

This is because babies are born relatively *insensitive* initially.

This helps to numb the discomfort of the birthing process for babies, and allows them to concentrate on establishing feeds and gaining weight.

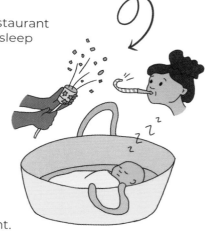

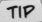 **TIP**

If you do take your newborn to a concert, make sure they have ear protection.

By 3–4 weeks, this insensitivity begins to wane and babies 'wake up', becoming more alert and unsettled by external stimuli. As well as being more responsive to external stimuli, they will no longer tolerate internal discomfort either.

This means we need to:

- employ settling techniques
- search for causes of discomfort and unsettled behaviour.

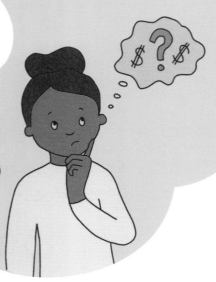

So, the million-dollar question: how do I settle a baby?

Return them to the womb

The more you understand this concept, the more easily you will be able to settle your baby. Think back to the moment in your life when you felt most relaxed. Was it while lying on the beach in the sun? Was it during a massage or a sleep-in? Sure, these things are relaxing, but life's demands are still waiting for you, just around the corner.

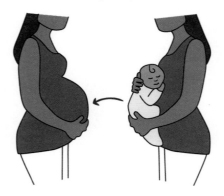

The truest answer to that question is when you were in utero, growing inside your mother's womb.

It's temperature controlled, nourishment is taken care of, there's no need for bathroom breaks, no mortgages, no bills to pay, no emails – not one iota of stress or anxiety.

Whenever a baby – or indeed someone at any age of life – is calmed, it's by using techniques that return them to that feeling of being inside the womb. These techniques are: shush, move, pat and swaddle and are fine to be used at any time in the first three weeks of life.

Shush

White noise or making a 'shush' sound loud enough that they are able to hear it.

Move

Swaying and rocking with your baby in your arms mimics the movements they felt in the womb. Movement such as the subtle bumps from a car ride or walk in the stroller will also help settle them.

Pat

This is the simplest, yet most poorly performed of the settling techniques. This is designed to remind your baby of the gentle tap of their mother's aorta (the main blood vessel) along their spine during pregnancy. Ignore any advice that the harder you pat the more settled they'll be! Patting should be slow – roughly one pat per second – and very gentle.

Swaddle

Swaddling your baby gives them a sense of security and calms their startle reflex. Try to alter their position, like holding your baby in your arms on their side or on their stomach.

See
pg. 130

Try using one or all of the above tools in unison. They're great ways to help calm your newborn baby.

Interestingly, it is no different when trying to comfort an older child, or even an adult. If you come across a person having a panic attack, you might see them rocking back and forth. We pat them or rub their back, say 'shhh' and hug them tight – **shush, move, pat, swaddle**. These manoeuvres calm all mammals at any age.

> **Regulate your own energy: calm yourself first. If you are not calm and relaxed yourself, it's near impossible to calm someone else.**

Babies are excellent communicators, remember – they drink much more than milk. They drink your warmth, your love, your connectedness. But they also drink your anxiety, your worry, your stress and your fear.

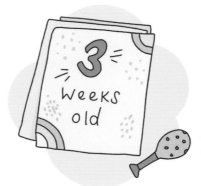

A baby's head rests directly on your bicep when being held. If you are tense, your muscles will tighten and your baby will sense this discomfort, imbibing it until they too, become stressed and unsettled.

If you're feeling overwhelmed, take a quiet break by yourself for five minutes. Make sure your baby is in a safe position, in a safe place, then take some time out. **Once composed, it's time to settle your baby.**

Remember, the shush, move, pat, swaddle techniques are fine to be used at any time in the first three weeks of life.

Beyond that, if you're relying on these techniques to get any peace and quiet, then there may be something that's being missed. After three weeks of life, a baby should be able to be cared for without relying on these settling manoeuvres all the time.

Note: Not using these techniques after three weeks of life isn't about being cruel or neglectful to our babies – quite the opposite. It's about ensuring that your baby's reliance on you isn't masking something that is driving their unsettled behaviour. If we don't try and understand what's causing their discomfort, we are doing our kids a disservice.

Dummies

In addition to the settling methods of shush, pat, move and swaddle, **sucking** is an innate soother and can be used in combination with other settling techniques. Using a dummy as a settling tool is perfectly okay; you could also put your clean little finger upside down in your baby's mouth to encourage them to suck.

Babies are born with an innate sucking reflex. Allowing them to suck helps activate their calming reflex, leading to more settled behaviour. If your baby remains unsettled after a feed and you are struggling to find a way to calm them, a dummy may provide the extra comfort needed.

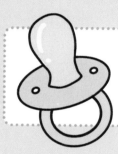

For breastfeeding infants, introducing a dummy early can affect attachment and supply, so it's best to wait until breastfeeding is properly established.

Dummies can be used briefly DURING the burping process (see page 166), but be careful not to overuse them, as this can potentially mask unsettled behaviour. Be mindful not to replace a feed with a dummy and make sure your baby is not using too much of their energy sucking on a non-food source.

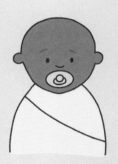

Safe sleep

The American Academy of Pediatrics and the Red Nose Foundation recommend room-sharing for the first 6–12 months of your baby's life, as this has been shown to reduce the risk of Sudden Infant Death Syndrome (SIDS). Room sharing also makes it easier for parents to comfort, feed and watch their baby.

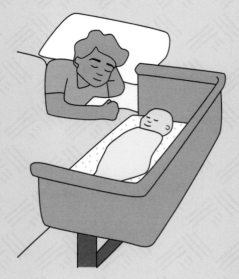

I'm a proud Red Nose Australia Ambassador, a not-for-profit organisation working on decreasing the risk of SIDS.

Visit rednose.org for more information.

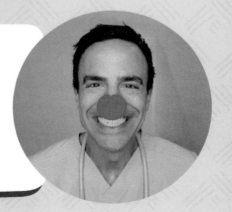

In addition to room-sharing early in life, here are four of the most important safe-sleeping tips.

1. Sleep baby on back

- Sleeping baby on the side or tummy increases the risk of SIDS.

2. Keep head and face uncovered

- Baby on back
- Feet to bottom of the cot
- Blankets tucked in firmly

- Use a safe baby sleeping bag with fitted neck, arm holes and no hood.

Covering a baby's head or face increases the risk of SIDS.

3. Keep baby smoke free before and after birth

Smoking during pregnancy and around your baby after birth increases the risk of SIDS. Help to quit smoking is available from your doctor, nurse or by contacting **Quitline in Australia on 13 7848.**

4. Ensure a safe sleeping environment night and day

- **Safe cot:** should meet the current standard in your country. Old cots will often not meet these standards.

- **Safe mattress:** firm, clean, flat and the right size for the cot.

- **Safe bedding:** soft surfaces and bulky bedding increase the risk of SIDS.

- **Temperature:** make sure your child is dressed appropriately for the temperature. See page 126 for temperature and TOG recommendations.

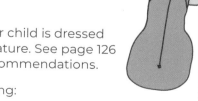

No soft surfaces or bulky bedding:

- ☒ pillow
- ☒ cot bumper
- ☒ lambswool
- ☒ soft toys
- ☒ doona or top sheets

Darkness

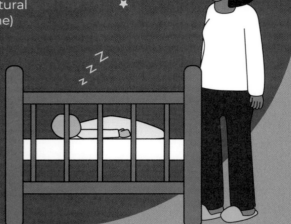

For the first 3–4 weeks after babies are born, they are quite insensitive to noise and light.

When combined with the residual melatonin (the body's natural sleep-promotion hormone) from their mother's placenta, which is still flowing through their system, they are usually happy to sleep in a light-filled room during the day.

But after 3–4 weeks, babies become increasingly sensitive, which means a darker room becomes important.

Melatonin production is increased in the absence of light. From about 3–4 weeks, making sure your baby's sleep environment is as dark as possible will help encourage that melatonin production. This will prevent cat-napping and help them learn to link their sleep cycles.

There are many block-out blinds available for purchase, including temporary ones that stick onto the window glass. If outside, darken the pram or portable bassinet with a **breathable blackout cover**. Don't use a blanket, as this doesn't usually provide enough darkness and the temperature can become dangerously high.

White noise

Most parents will tell you that their baby sleeps more soundly when the vacuum is going, or the washing machine is on.

Babies LOVE white (background) noise, and it can become a very positive sleep association for your baby.

Why is white noise so soothing for babies?

If we consider the concept of the fourth trimester, this helps us to understand where the most effective settling techniques are derived from. The different measures we discussed earlier (shush, move, pat and swaddle) which essentially return our babies to the feeling of being in the womb, are extremely effective.

Now think about what a baby hears when in the womb – it's similar to being under water. This is the theory behind using white noise as a settling technique.

When we remind babies of that time in the womb with shushing noises or white noise machines, they settle further, and this helps to link their sleep cycles. It also drowns out other household or environmental noise, such as traffic or dogs barking.

White noise should be used as early as possible, as this will teach your baby to associate it with sleep time.

I love white noise because it is inexpensive, easy and portable.

There are many free apps available that create these sounds, but this can be highly annoying if your phone is stuck with the sleeping baby, so I recommend a portable or and plug-in white noise machine.

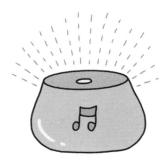

Some common questions about white noise include:

 What level should I play it at?

White noise should be played at a medium level (around the volume level of a shower running) and when your baby is crying, it can be turned up so they can hear it over their cries, then turned down when they're calm and settled. It should be played for every sleep, for the entire duration of sleep, even overnight. It's amazing how many parents tell me their own sleep has benefited too!

Protecting little ears is important – see my notes on page 203 for more on this.

See pg. 203

 When should you stop using white noise?

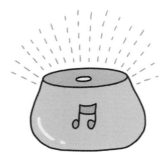

It's perfectly safe to continue to use white noise throughout childhood and adolescence, but if you do want to start weaning your toddler or child off it, then simply turn it down bit by bit every night until they no longer need it.

What do all the other colour noises mean?

More recently, research has popped up regarding different forms of white noise, including pink, brown and black.

 WHITE noise covers all audible frequencies of sound.

 PINK noise is deeper, like a bass rumble. Rain or a heartbeat are examples of pink noise, with a deeper feel to it.

 BROWN noise moves deeper still, like the sound of a waterfall continually crashing, or a deep rumbling of thunder.

 BLACK noise is the exact opposite – an absence of sound, like one would hear in outer space. Some adults prefer absolute silence to sleep in, but babies often find this quite disconcerting.

Of all the background noise colours and frequencies, white noise is the only one that has research to support it, in terms of paediatric sleep ... but you may find that as your baby grows into a toddler, they prefer brown/nature sounds – it's what I prefer now!

 Won't my baby get addicted to white noise?

The short answer is YES ... but the long one is that it doesn't matter.

As discussed above, it's inexpensive, easy and portable.

Room temperature and dressing

The ideal room temperature for a baby is between 19°C and 22°C (66–72°F).

Babies commonly wake in the early hours of the morning because they are cold.

Dressing your baby appropriately is the key to ensuring both safety and a good night's sleep. Your baby cannot regulate their temperature like adults, so it is important to ensure they are safe and comfortable.

Thermal Overall Grade (TOG)

Thermal Overall Grade (TOG) is a measure of the insulation and warmth of sleepwear and bedding. The lower the **TOG rating**, the lighter the fabric. The higher the rating, the more padded it is, and the more suitable it is for cooler temperatures. When buying sleepwear like swaddles, sleeping bags, sleep suits or bedding, look for **TOG-rated** products. These are most helpful, and more precise than something simply being labelled a 'winter weight' or 'summer weight' product.

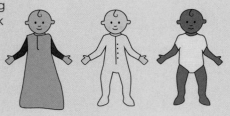

Bedroom temperature	Clothing	Swaddle/ sleeping bag	Blanket
19–22°C	Singlet and long-sleeve/ long-leg onesie	2.5 TOG bag	Optional
23–24°C	Long-sleeve/ long-leg onesie	1.0 TOG bag	No
25+°C	Short-sleeve/sleeveless bodysuit or just a nappy	0.2 TOG bag	No

Co-sleeping

Co-sleeping is different to room-sharing; it's bed-sharing, and it's important to state upfront that co-sleeping can be dangerous and has been shown to increase the risk of SIDS.

With that said, in some cultures co-sleeping is very common, and in my experience as a paediatrician, co-sleeping eventuates more commonly in the setting of an unsettled baby.

If you choose to co-sleep, it's important that you:

1. know how to practise co-sleeping safely.

2. understand that it can make it harder for your child to learn to sleep independently.

See pg. 126

If you're intending to establish a routine around the six-week mark and have your baby sleeping independently during the day, this can be much more difficult if you co-sleep at night.

When making this decision, the most important thing is doing what feels right for your family.

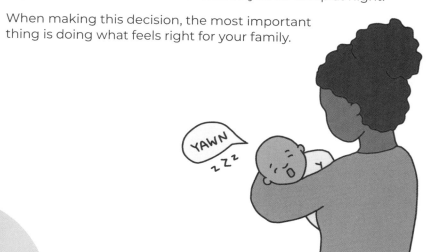

Co-sleeping guidelines

If you plan to co-sleep with your baby, Red Nose Australia recommends the following guidelines:

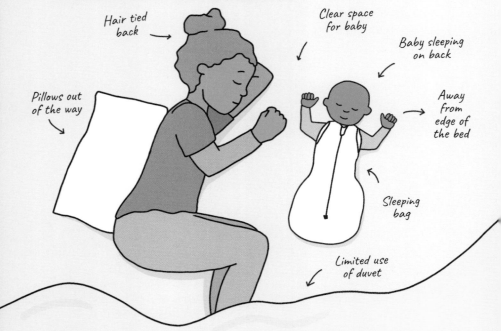

Hair tied back →

Clear space for baby ↓

Baby sleeping on back ↘

Pillows out of the way ↘

Away from edge of the bed →

Sleeping bag ↖

Limited use of duvet ↙

(**1.**) **Place your baby on their back to sleep.**

Never place your baby on their tummy or side.
This helps to protect their airway.

(**2.**) **Keep baby's head and face uncovered.**

Keep pillows and adult bedding away from your baby.

Use a safe sleeping bag with no hood and with baby's arms out.

Don't wrap or swaddle baby when
bed-sharing or co-sleeping.

(**3.**) **Make sure the mattress is firm and flat.**

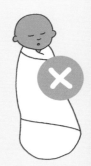

Don't use a waterbed, or anything soft underneath,
such as a lambswool underlay or pillows. These can
increase the risk of overheating and suffocation.

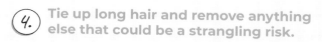

4. Tie up long hair and remove anything else that could be a strangling risk.

This includes all jewellery, teething necklaces and dummy chains.

5. Move the bed away from the wall.

This ensures your baby can't get trapped between the bed and the wall.

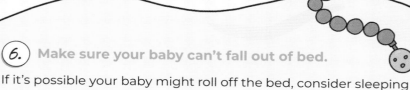

6. Make sure your baby can't fall out of bed.

If it's possible your baby might roll off the bed, consider sleeping on your mattress on the floor.

7. Create a clear space for your baby.

Place your baby on their back to the side of one parent, away from the edge.

Never position your baby in between two adults or next to other children or pets, as this can increase the risk of overheating and suffocation.

· ·

You should never co-sleep or lie down while holding a baby if:

· you are overly tired or unwell
· you or your partner have recently consumed alcohol
· you or your partner smoke, even if you don't smoke in the bedroom
· you or your partner have taken any medications that make you feel sleepy or less aware
· baby is premature or small for their gestational age.

Note: Falling asleep while holding a baby on a couch or chair is always unsafe. Move yourself and your baby to a safe sleep environment if you think you might fall asleep.

Importance of swaddling

Swaddling is an integral part of the settling process.

This warm, enveloping hug returns babies to the feeling of being snug in a warm, tight womb – and **forms a fundamental part of the calming method. Here I'll show you two foolproof techniques for achieving the perfect wrap.**

There is a second reason why a tight swaddle improves sleep and settling. Beyond resembling a warm hug, the swaddle is also there to limit your baby's **startle reflex.**

The startle reflex is also called the **Moro – or parachute – reflex,** where your baby will suddenly throw their arms and legs out when startled, or even spontaneously, without trigger. It's sometimes referred to as the **parachute reflex**, because the baby looks like they're jumping out of an aeroplane and preparing to launch their parachute. This sudden jolt of movement can often wake a baby, or give them such a shock that they begin to cry.

Swaddling limits the baby's arm movement to minimise this shock. But always remember: the arms can be swaddled, but never swaddle the legs too. This is to protect the hips – more on this shortly.

Note: Once your baby starts to roll (usually around the four month mark) you'll need to unswaddle them.

Which style of swaddle to pick?

Your baby will have adopted a particular position in the womb.

Many parents will remember that during scans, their baby's hands were always up covering their face, by their sides or across their chest. Either way, try to replicate this posture – this is likely to be the most successful swaddle position for your baby.

Traditional wrap swaddle

The **traditional wrap** is just that – a standard, traditional wrap that suits most babies. Here, the arms are folded across the chest or abdomen.

This technique will keep your baby's hands well away from their face, and is particularly useful for babies:

See
pg. 156

- who have a strong or disruptive rooting reflex (trying to suck on anything, including their hands – see page 156 for more on this).

- who suffer from eczema (dry skin), as keeping fingernails away from an itchy face is crucial.

Angel wrap swaddle

The **angel wrap** is a great swaddling technique to achieve a hands-up position, or for babies who like to suck on their hands or their swaddle to self-soothe. It allows a small degree of movement, but not enough to trigger the rooting or Moro reflexes, and prevents face scratching. It is a modified traditional wrap with one crucial initial step – creating a collar.

Traditional wrap:

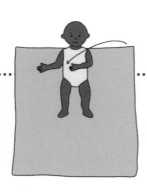

Step 1: Use a large muslin wrap or stretch jersey material. The bigger the better. Lay it flat in a square shape.

Step 2: Take your baby and lie them in the middle of the wrap with their head above the top edge of the material.

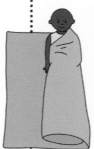

Step 3: Bring one of their arms across their body so it sits above their belly button.

Step 4: Wrap that side of the material across their folded arm and tuck it firmly underneath the other side of their body.

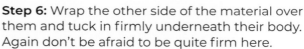

Step 5: Bring their other arm across their body so both arms are folded above their belly button.

Step 6: Wrap the other side of the material over them and tuck in firmly underneath their body. Again don't be afraid to be quite firm here.

Step 7: Open the bottom part of the wrap so it makes a triangle shape.

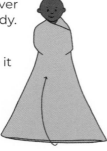

Step 8: Bring it up over your baby and tuck it loosely around their body, ensuring the material doesn't come above their chest.

Remember: **For both styles of wrap, firm over the shoulders, loose over the hips.**

Angel wrap:

Step 1: Use a large muslin wrap or stretch jersey material, the bigger the better. Lay it flat in a square shape.

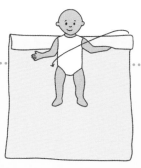

Step 2: This part is the crucial bit: fold about 10 centimetres of material over at the top of the wrap.

Step 3: Take your baby and lie them in the middle of the wrap with their head above the top edge of the material, like the collar of a shirt.

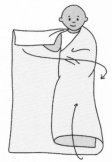

Step 4: Take one of your baby's arms and bring it up next to their shoulder, tucking their hand up under the folded part of the material.

Step 5: Bring that side of the material across their body and tuck it underneath the other side of them. Don't be afraid to be firm here.

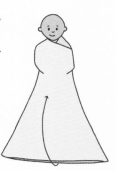

Step 6: Repeat on the other side with the other arm.

Step 7: Wrap the other side of the material over them and tuck it in firmly underneath, using their body weight to keep it in place.

Step 8: Open the bottom part of the wrap so it makes a triangle shape.

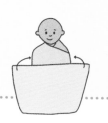

Step 9: Bring it up over your baby and tuck it loosely around their body, ensuring the material doesn't come above their chest.

Safe swaddling/wrapping

Tips to allow for natural hip development during swaddling/wrapping

DOs

- ☑ Position your baby with their hips bent and knees apart in a frog position.
- ☑ Allow enough room, from the waist down, for free leg movement (a triangle shape is a good guide).
- ☑ Swaddle the upper body firmly, but not tightly.
- ☑ Swaddle the arms only.
- ☑ Follow SIDS guidelines.
- ☑ Stop swaddling once your baby is rolling.

DON'Ts

- ☒ Swaddle legs tightly or straight down/ pressed together.
- ☒ Use sleep sacks or pouches that are snug around the thighs.

Note: Incorrect swaddling techniques can increase the risk of hip dysplasia. It is important to swaddle your baby's arms but leave the legs to 'flop open'. This encourages the hips to mature. **Always remember: firm top half, loose bottom half.**

Baby carriers

When my first baby was on the way, one of the items at the top of my list to buy was a carrier. I love carriers, particularly in the early days/weeks. They keep our babies close to us, upright (if your baby is colicky, they'll love this) and, most importantly, they keep your hands free!

There are many different types and styles, and everyone has their own preference. In the first four weeks, I love the stretchy body wraps that are tied around you.

Once your baby is larger/heavier you'll probably need a more structured carrier to protect your back and keep your baby comfortable. I recommend a carrier with padded shoulders and adjustable waist bands, so it's easy to share between parents.

When using a carrier, there are two key things to remember:

Healthy hip positioning

- Correct hip positioning means your baby's:
  - hips are spread so their legs straddle your body
  - knees are spread apart
  - thighs are supported
  - hips are bent.
- This encourages healthy hip development.
- If your baby is at high risk of hip dysplasia, time in the carrier is often recommended to help reduce the risk.

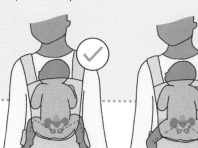

2. Use the **T.I.C.K.S.** rule to position your baby safely in a sling or carrier and avoid suffocation risks.

 Tight:

- The sling or carrier should be tight, with the baby positioned high and upright with head support.
- Any loose fabric might cause your baby to slump down, which could restrict breathing.

In view at all times:

- You should always be able to see your baby's face by simply looking down.
- Ensure your baby's face, nose and mouth remain uncovered by the sling and/or your body.

 Close enough to kiss:

- Your baby should be close enough to your chin that by tipping their head forward, you can easily kiss it.
- You can purchase newborn insert cushions for many carriers which will help keep your baby at the correct (kissable) height.

 Keep chin off the chest:

- Ensure your baby's chin is up and away from their body.
- Your baby should never be curled so that their chin is forced onto their chest. This can restrict breathing.
- Regularly check your baby as babies can be in distress without making any noice or movement.

 Supported back:

- Your baby's back should be supported in a natural position with their tummy and chest against you.
- When bending over, support your baby with one hand behind their back.
- Bend at the knees, not at the waist.

Hip health

When it comes to swaddling and settling babies, we talk a lot about hip health. The hip joint is a ball-and-socket joint that allows an incredible range of movement without much risk of dislocation (unlike the shoulder).

When babies are born, the socket is very shallow, and doesn't hold the ball particularly tight. The socket matures over time, and most babies develop a nice, stable hip joint without any intervention required.

But one in six newborns have some ongoing hip instability, and incorrect swaddling techniques can increase the risk of hip dysplasia.

What is hip dysplasia?

Hip dysplasia is a common condition that occurs when the ball and socket of the hip do not fit together in their 'normal' position. When the socket fails to mature properly and remains shallow, this leaves the hip joint vulnerable, and increases the risk of early-onset arthritis. This is the most common cause of hip arthritis in adults. Imagine needing a hip replacement in your thirties – not fun.

Early diagnosis of hip dysplasia optimises treatment outcomes, but prevention is even better.

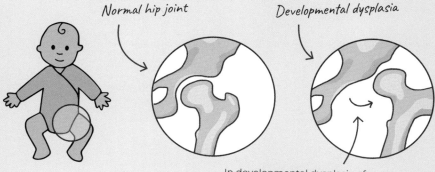

Normal hip joint

Developmental dysplasia

In developmental dysplasia of the hip, the ball part of the joint can come out of the socket.

Risk factors for hip dysplasia include:

- being female (hip dysplasia affects girls more than boys)
- being the firstborn
- a family history of hip dysplasia
- being breech during pregnancy
- being a multiple (twin, triplet etc.)
- a neuromuscular or connective tissue disorder
- inappropriate swaddling.

Signs and symptoms of hip dysplasia:

- a 'clunk' or 'click' when moving hip during an examination. (Be aware that many parts of a baby's lower limb can click when moved; this sound is not necessarily emanating from the hip. A hip assessment should be done by a professional.)
- uneven thigh creases
- crooked buttock creases
- difficulty in spreading legs apart when changing nappies
- weight off to one side when sitting
- different leg lengths
- avoiding weight bearing in an older baby
- walking on tippy toes on one side
- limping when walking
- metatarsus adductus (abnormal foot position).

Every child's hips need checking at the following intervals to ensure they're developing appropriately:

- birth
- 1–4 weeks
- 6–8 weeks
- 6–9 months
- 12 months
- Then at the usual health reviews until 3.5 years.

Your doctor will examine your baby's hips and determine if an ultrasound is required to measure the degree of hip maturity.

BATHS

Baths can create a wind-down routine and sleep association

Remember that an essential part of settling a baby is to return them to the feeling of being in the womb. A nice warm bath is a beautiful example of that feeling – **so bath time should not be dreaded by parents.** It shouldn't be a messy, hurried chore, **but rather a calming time for both baby and parent.**

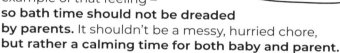

It's okay to bath your baby every 2–3 days at home. **Bathing every day is not necessary in the newborn period.**

Once you're trying to establish a rhythm, a bath can become a lovely part of an evening wind-down routine, providing benefits to both you and your baby.

Baths should be calming and relaxing, and avoided when your baby is overtired or too hungry. Make sure you don't delay sleeps or feeds just to fit in a bath. After your baby's bath, a couple of lullabies, a feed and cuddle are all you need to complete a simple evening wind-down routine for your baby.

If you follow this routine regularly, your baby will learn to anticipate bedtime. This can help your baby settle for the night and create a wonderful association with sleep onset – one that can last a lifetime.

Being organised at bath time is the key to success

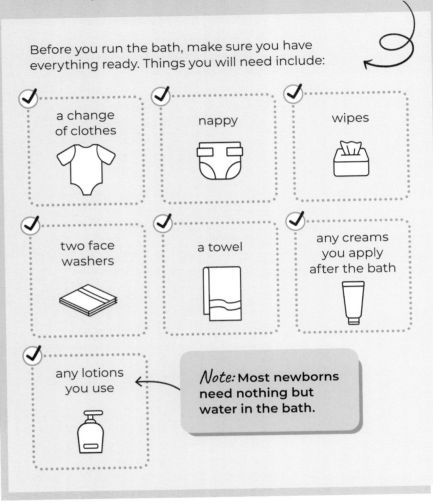

Before you run the bath, make sure you have everything ready. Things you will need include:

☑ a change of clothes

☑ nappy

☑ wipes

☑ two face washers

☑ a towel

☑ any creams you apply after the bath

☑ any lotions you use

Note: Most newborns need nothing but water in the bath.

Note: If you're breastfeeding after bath time, make sure you've got your pillow, drink bottle and phone (whatever you need) ready to go, so it's a seamless transition. I often recommend half a feed (half a bottle or one breast) before the bath and half after. Remember, it is very difficult to calmly bathe a hungry baby.

Treat bath time like a day spa

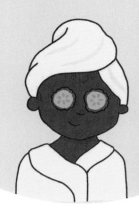

Start by ensuring the bathroom is warm and that your hands are not icy cold.

It's very unpleasant for a baby to be undressed and feel cold and unswaddled, and if they enter the bath screaming, it's hard to achieve that nice, calm state.

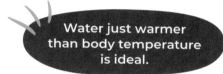

Water just warmer than body temperature is ideal.

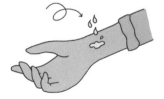

The temperature of the bath can have a big impact on how enjoyable the experience is. When you run the water, test it with your inner wrist instead of your fingertips. Your wrist is more sensitive to temperature. If the water is too hot for your wrist, it's too hot for your baby.

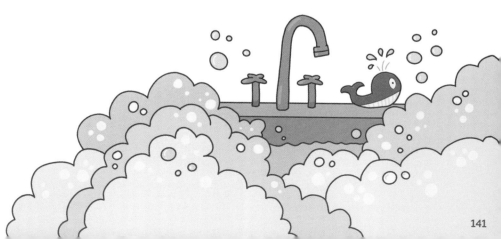

Seven simple steps to the perfect baby bath

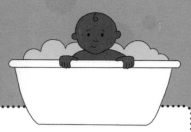

Step 1: Get everything ready as described, then fill the bath. If choosing to share a bath with your baby, ensure another person is available to help get them out at the end.

Step 2: Undress your baby and ease them into the bath, resting their neck on your wrist and holding them under their armpit with your thumb and index finger. This will free up your second hand and create a firm, safe hold.

Step 3: Wet one of the face washers and place it over your baby's tummy. This provides extra warmth and a feeling of security, as well as dampening their startle (Moro) reflex. Remember to frequently tip water over the face washer, as it will become cold when not submerged.

Step 4: Start at the top and wash their face with the other wet face washer. Be sure to clean underneath their neck creases and behind their ears. Soap is seldom required. If your baby is comfortable, you can trickle water over their face. This will help get them comfortable in water and prepare them for swimming at a later age.

Step 5: Move down their body, washing their bottom last, then dispose of that face washer. Don't keep a newborn in the bath for too long – a few minutes is all they need.

Step 6: Lift the baby out of the bath and straight onto a clean, dry towel. Try to keep them warm as you pat them dry, ensuring you've dried all the creases and crevices, such as under their chin and under their armpits, as well as the groin. These are the main places at risk of becoming irritated and developing a rash if not dried properly. Use this opportunity to sing, smile or babble with your baby – these are small moments of magic!

Step 7: Apply any creams you are using and then a new nappy, followed by their clothes or sleep suit and swaddles.

Rashes (and other completely normal things in the first few weeks of life)

Erythema toxicum/ newborn acne

Erythema toxicum (or toxic erythema), also known as newborn acne, is the most common rash in the first few days or weeks of a baby's life. It seldom occurs in premature babies. The cause is similar to that of pimples in adolescence, with wild hormone fluctuations after birth and during breastfeeding leading to pimples.

Newborn acne does not appear on the palms of the hands or the soles of the feet. It's not painful or itchy, and doesn't cause scarring. The spots are scattered red, with white centres. Sometimes pustules can also be present, in a severe form of toxic erythema called transient neonatal pustular melanosis. This typically occurs with darker skinned babies, and is also harmless.

Miliaria

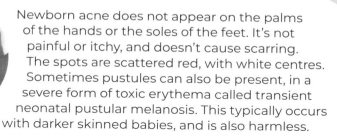

Miliaria is a rash caused by blockages in the small sweat ducts. This commonly occurs on the forehead, neck and upper chest in newborns (miliaria crystallina). Sometimes the blockages can be deeper in the skin and become red too; this is called miliaria rubra (when red). It's essentially a heat rash and resolves when the child is made cooler and more comfortable.

Milia

Milia is a rash that affects more than half of newborn babies. It has the appearance of hundreds of tiny white dots, mostly seen on the nose. This is due to an accumulation of sweat and old skin cells in blocked pores. It resolves within the first month of life.

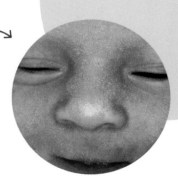

When these accumulations occur inside the mouth, they're called Bohn nodules (roof of the mouth) and Epstein pearls (margin of the gum). It's easy to mistake these for neonatal teeth, so speak to your doctor if you're not sure.

Sucking blisters

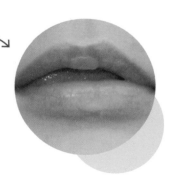

Sucking blisters are commonly seen on newborns' lips, due to vigorous sucking at the breast or bottle. They are firm swellings, as opposed to fluid-filled, and resolve without any treatment.

Cutis marmorata

Cutis marmorata means *mottled skin*, and refers to the lace-like appearance of skin that occurs in some newborns. It's symmetrical on both sides of the body and is the skin's response to cold. Newborn babies haven't yet had to control their body temperature, thanks to the luxury of a nine-month temperature-controlled bath, so after birth they sometimes struggle with adapting to the cold and to constant changes in environmental temperature. This can generally be resolved by gently warming the skin. Cutis marmorata can continue to affect children well into older childhood.

Acrocyanosis

Acrocyanosis means blue/purple hands and feet. When isolated to the extremities it is of no concern, and occurs because these parts are the most likely to be cold, being the furthest from the child's heart. Acrocyanosis is always most dramatic immediately after birth and following a bath.

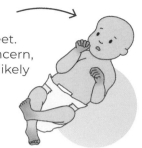

Breast changes

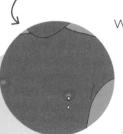

White nipple discharge, also called witch's milk, can occur in both girls and boys. Breastfeeding mothers pass a breastfeeding hormone called prolactin to babies via their milk which stimulates the baby to make milk, too. High circulating oestrogen in a pregnant woman causes the breast tissue to enlarge (gynaecomastia); it can also result in vaginal discharge in baby girls.

Cradle cap

Cradle cap is a very common skin condition affecting the baby's scalp, and usually disappears by three months of age. Symptoms range from subtle dandruff-like flakes to thick, yellow crusting throughout the scalp. It can also appear in the eyebrows.

Cradle cap is never itchy or painful, and applying moisturiser won't help. Infected cradle cap is uncommon, but if your child seems unwell, develops a fever or their scalp becomes smelly, see a doctor.

Although moisturiser won't fix it, applying moisturiser or oil to the flakes can loosen them and enable you to lift them off using your nails or a fine-toothed comb. I recommend simply using olive oil and combing off the flakes during bath time.

Anti-dandruff shampoos can also be helpful for difficult-to-clear cases, but don't use these for more than two weeks, as they can dry or irritate the scalp.

Eczema

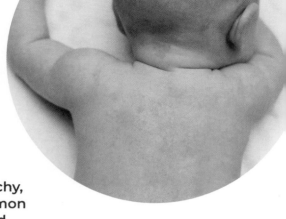

Eczema – or atopic dermatitis – is a skin condition that causes dry, red and scaly skin almost anywhere on the body. Eczema is extremely itchy, and is a relatively common contributor to unsettled infant behaviour.

If severe, the dry skin will eventually start to crack and bleed, leading to a risk of infection.

At what age do kids get eczema?

Eczema commonly starts in the first months of life, and often gets missed, as it can resemble newborn acne. The key difference is that with eczema, the skin is very dry to touch, almost like sandpaper. In the case of mild eczema, most children will outgrow the condition by the age of five years. Certain things can cause flares of eczema, such as allergens (food, pet hair, pollen, etc.), excessive heat, stress or having a cold.

Eczema can run in the family

Eczema tends to occur in families, especially when there is a history of atopy – a tendency to sensitivity, such as eczema, asthma, allergy or hayfever. If either parent has ever had eczema, there is an 80 per cent chance their child will be affected too.

The number one enemy of eczema is heat!

Given that eczema is essentially extreme dryness, the number one enemy of eczema is heat. To prevent overheating, try removing a single layer (clothing or blanket) from your baby, while also ensuring your baby never gets too cold. Clothing made of natural fibres and breathable fabric is preferable. Regular moisturising helps to return moisture to the dry skin and, occasionally, medicated creams/ointments may also be needed; discuss this with your child's doctor.

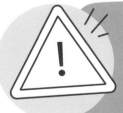

Never rub food on your baby's skin, especially in babies with eczema, as this may increase the chance of your baby developing a food allergy. Always wash your hands after eating if your baby has eczema.

Positional plagiocephaly (flat head syndrome)

Positional plagiocephaly (play-jee-oh-KEF-uh-lee) is also referred to as flat head syndrome. This is usually the result of sleeping babies on their backs in the first months of life – something we do to reduce the risk of SIDS, and should never be avoided.

Signs of plagiocephaly:

- The back of the baby's head is flatter on one side.
- The baby usually has less hair on that part of their head.
- When looking down at the baby's head from above, the forehead on the flattened side may look pushed forward and asymmetric.

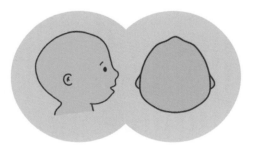

Normocephalic: this is a medical term for normal head shape.

Brachycephaly: this is a form of plagiocephaly where the back of the head may be symmetric, but is quite flat, instead of normally rounded.

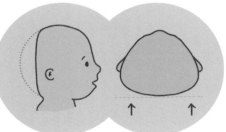

Unilateral plagiocephaly: this occurs when pressure is applied to one side of the back of the head. It flattens this part and as it progressively worsens, causes the same side to protrude forward at the front (the face).

How to prevent/treat plagiocephaly:

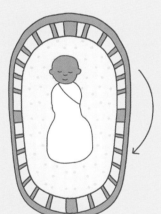

- Tummy time!
- Repositioning manoeuvres e.g. ensuring your baby doesn't favour looking to one side with every sleep. This can be done by moving their head once they fall into a deep sleep.

- If your baby always turns their head towards you, move the bassinet to another place or rotate your baby's position with each sleep, so their head is at the top of the bassinet one night and at the bottom the next night, etc.

- If your baby can't move their head due to neck stiffness, this needs to be reviewed by a doctor or paediatric physiotherapist.

- Time – the stronger the baby gets, the less time they spend on their backs, allowing their head to naturally reconfigure, up until the age of two years.

In severe cases, a doctor may prescribe a helmet. Helmets make the head rounder more quickly. But, on average, studies have shown that after a couple of years, babies who don't get helmets usually have similar results to those with helmets.

TRANSLATING YOUR BABY

Not every squawk or movement that comes from a baby is a sign of hunger. Babies have different ways of communicating hunger, tiredness and wind.

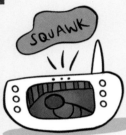

Our babies are incredible non-verbal communicators, and it is our job to learn to read their cues. There are myriad reasons why babies cry excessively, from wind to illness, hunger to eczema, being overtired or hot and everything in between.

When it comes to identifying the cause of a baby's unsettled behaviour, parental instinct has been shown to correlate strongly with the true cause. The better you understand your baby's cues, the better you will be at interpreting their needs and deciphering their messages.

My entire philosophy is designed to turn the volume up on that innate parental instinct and empower you to understand your baby better.

Hunger signs

While not every movement or noise from a baby will be a sign of hunger, it's important to feed your baby when you do see hunger signs. If you miss these hunger signs, then your baby will become more unsettled and upset, which can make it very difficult to calm and feed them. They will latch at the breast more easily (or take a bottle more calmly) if you start the feed when they first show hunger signs.

Your baby is looking for a feed if they are:

searching for a breast or bottle

opening their mouth

licking their lips

beginning to cry in short bursts.

It's possible to recognise early, middle and late cues for hunger.

**Early cues:
'I'm hungry'**

- Rooting and turning towards the breast or bottle.
- Stirring from being asleep.
- Mouth opening.

**Mid cues:
'I'm really hungry'**

- Bringing their hand to their mouth.
- Stretching and increasing physical movement.
- Sticking out their tongue or licking their lips and making sucking noises.

**Late cues:
'Calm me first, then feed me'**

- Crying.
- Agitated body movements.
- Colour – face turning red.

Tired signs

Tired signs generally occur within one hour of your newborn being awake. Rather than strictly watching the clock, watch your baby closely for any of these signs and, once observed, begin soothing your baby and put them down for a nap. This is the optimal time for a baby to fall asleep, and will prevent them from becoming overtired.

What happens if our baby gets overtired?

While the aim is to get our babies ready for sleep when we see those initial tired signs, in reality, it's not always possible. From time to time (for many reasons) they'll move past the 'I'm ready for bed phase' and into the 'overtired phase'.

Once this happens they will be very **hard to settle and struggle to fall asleep independently**. If you're at this stage, you'll need to use your settling techniques (swaddling, rocking, patting, white noise) to help calm your baby and help them fall asleep – they may need an assisted nap.

Assisted naps are exactly that – they're naps where your baby has some assistance from you to sleep.

Your baby may sleep:

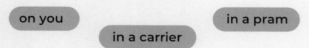

on you   in a carrier   in a pram

Remember – just like the settling techniques – assisted naps are fine to be used every now and then but if you're relying on them for every sleep, something is being missed and this needs to be investigated.

I'm getting tired

More vocal and chatting

Distant looks/stares

Appearing bored

Red eyebrows/eyelids

Starts posseting/spilling milk more despite not being fed for some time

Jerky movements

I'm ready for bed

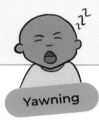

Yawning

Eye rubbing

Pulling hair/ears

Wanting to suck and appearing hungry

Grizzling

Making fists with hands

I'm overtired

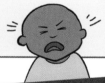

Back-arching

Hysterical crying

Stiff body

Very difficult to settle

Wind signs

**Trapped wind is incredibly uncomfortable for babies –
I talk about this in depth in on page 158.**

The single most common mistake I see with parents
of newborns is the **misinterpreting of wind signs**.

Unsettled babies who cry a lot will often be **dismissed
as hungry** – especially by onlookers, who'll tell you
you're not feeding them enough! There's also the desire
to feed just to stop the crying. A baby crying can be
unbelievably distressing for both baby and parent.

The human brain is designed to be
exquisitely sensitive to the sound of a
baby's cry – it's something we're built
to NOT withstand. This is an excellent
protective measure, an innate reflex
that ensures we pay close attention
to the safety and needs of our baby.

**It's little wonder elite military units
train themselves to withstand
extreme stresses, things like
sleep deprivation, hunger, loud
noises – sounds just like having
a newborn, doesn't it?!**

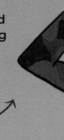

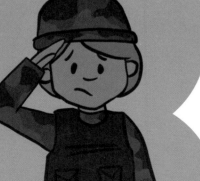

Wind signs:

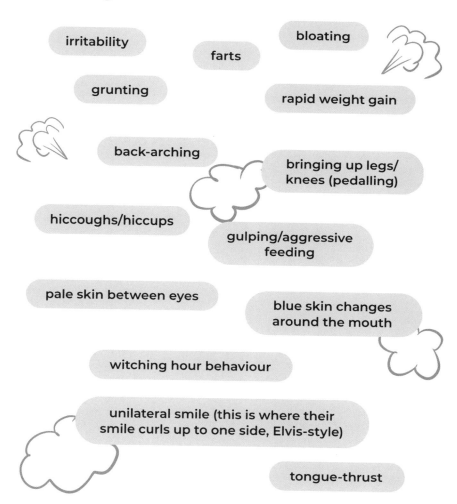

irritability

farts

bloating

grunting

rapid weight gain

back-arching

bringing up legs/knees (pedalling)

hiccoughs/hiccups

gulping/aggressive feeding

pale skin between eyes

blue skin changes around the mouth

witching hour behaviour

unilateral smile (this is where their smile curls up to one side, Elvis-style)

tongue-thrust

All these, together with **frequent feeding**, are clear signs that your baby is **not burping enough**, and will benefit from more burps with each feed. You should only feed in response to hunger, not in response to a different cause of discomfort or crying. When in doubt – burp more! See the section on active burping (page 162) for the best burping method.

Be careful not to misinterpret reflexes as signs of hunger

There are certain innate reflexes in a baby that can be activated, regardless of whether they are hungry or not.

Two examples of these are:

 1. **The Rooting Reflex**

- The rooting reflex is triggered by brushing your child's cheek, which triggers them to move their mouth towards that stimulus.

- If it is a breast or bottle, they will try to find it, and that might give you the impression that they're hungry.

- This is NOT always the case – remember, reflexes are just that: reflexive.

2. **The Sucking Reflex**

- When a baby is full and uncomfortable from excess wind, they might give the impression of being hungry, and root for a breast or bottle, then instantly start sucking when they find it. This causes parents and caregivers to think 'they must have just been hungry' – but this is absolutely wrong!

- They'll suck on a bottle, on your finger, on a dummy – they'll even suck on their fingers or their own tongue!

- This does not necessarily mean they want more milk – it is a reflex they can't turn off.

Note: We talk about these and other developmental reflexes in more depth on page 201.

Other hurdles that drive unsettled behaviour

This is a bit of a mental checklist that I suggest parents refer to when their baby is crying. The more we think holistically about our baby's comfort or discomfort, the more we can help identify, and eliminate, what's driving their unsettled behaviour.

Trapped wind

Room temperature

Room too light

Overtiredness

Eczema

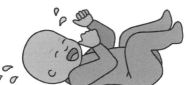
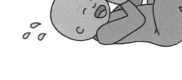

Intolerances

Hunger

Car or pram stopping

Tag on clothing itching them

Loud or abrupt noises waking them

Dirty nappy

Wind causes

Babies are 'obligate nose breathers'.

This means they prefer breathing through their nose, so that they can breathe while they feed. That's why our nostrils are shaped the way they are – to create a window for airflow, even when pressed against a breast.

This means that swallowing air is inevitable. It cannot be prevented, only corrected after the feed. This swallowed air needs to come out via burping, not out the other end, which will cause a series of very predictable problems.

> **Some people will tell you that you don't need to burp a newborn. This is incorrect.**

All babies need to burp, from the moment they start to feed. Not all will be deeply unsettled because of wind, especially in the first three weeks of life, but as they 'wake up' at 3–4 weeks, they can become increasingly bothered by it.

As discussed, in the first few days of life, newborns are often quite relaxed. They can be taken out to restaurants, movies, even a rock concert – and they will sleep soundly. This is because they are **relatively insensitive to stimuli.** This **includes internal stimuli.**

So, newborns don't suffer any less from wind, they just aren't sensitive to the pain yet.

By week three, and sometimes earlier, they are far more sensitive and will not tolerate residual wind. This can lead to unsettled behaviours and often frequent feeding, which creates a negative cycle: feeding traps wind, wind causes pain, pain causes crying and crying prompts a feed. So the cycle continues ...

Because we breathe while drinking, there's **no option but to swallow air.** This is called **aerophagia.**

This causes **problems NOW** and **LATER.**

The problems NOW:

1. **Your baby can feel full of air, not milk**

The stomach is the key here – at capacity, it stretches, which fires special receptors that tell the brain that it's time to stop eating. So, with a seemingly full stomach, often after only one breast or just a small volume via bottle, the baby will be satisfied.

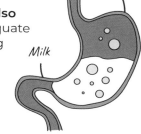

Air

Milk

Your baby is now half full of milk but also half full of air. This doesn't provide adequate sustenance until the next feed, meaning the baby will **feed more frequently.**

Feeding more frequently means the baby is getting less sleep, which they need to grow and develop.

2. **Frequent possets, spills and 'refluxed' milk**

Overstretching the stomach also leads to more frequent possets, which is why so many people get confused with a diagnosis of reflux. **Refluxed milk** is not the same as gastro-oesophageal reflux disease; these two terms are often used interchangeably, causing much distress. Refluxed milk is simply milk that travels backwards from the stomach to the mouth.

As the stretched stomach muscle tries to return to its regular size, your baby will invariably bring up some milk. Refluxed milk is common. We will discuss the overdiagnosis of reflux on page 184, as true reflux only affects a very small number of babies.

stomach returning to normal size

3. Lying down can become painful

Have you ever tried lying flat on a full stomach, or withholding a burp at your in-laws' house because you don't want to embarrass yourself at the table? It's uncomfortable and painful, and feels like a grenade is going off inside your chest.

This is why babies often show significant signs of discomfort immediately after a feed. Many parents tell me that their baby sleeps beautifully upright after a feed, but wakes immediately if they try to put them down.

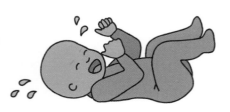

The problems LATER:

1. Your baby will need to fart to get rid of the trapped wind

Residual wind needs to move somewhere – it doesn't simply disappear. As the wind travels from the stomach to the small intestine, the baby begins to experience pain and discomfort.

Hours after a feed, that wind will make its way to the large intestine, where it **eventually becomes a fart.**

The movement through the large intestine is very uncomfortable, because the colon was designed to contract and squeeze on solid content, not wind. This is what frequently causes unsettled behaviour hours after the offending feed.

Farting may provide instant relief from wind, but the next wind bubble is just around the corner, causing more distress.

It is normal for a baby to fart, just like anyone. But too much farting is a sign of many missed burps.

Farting

We don't talk about it much (although of course it's very natural), but farting is actually really complicated!

You need to squeeze some muscles, relax other ones, make sure it is 'just' a fart – and coordinate all this at the same time. Understandably, babies struggle to do this!

They will feel a build-up of gas and then just flex every muscle they have, go red in the face and eventually pass wind – because it's the only valve that can blow.

 Cramping and pain

We have an innate reflex called the gastro-colic reflex, which causes the large intestine to begin contracting as soon as food enters the stomach. This is designed to propel poo out, to make room for what is coming. It's a genius design. However, when the large intestine contracts on gas – something it is not designed to do – this causes cramping and pain.

Babies with trapped wind feed well for the first part of a feed, but then arch their back and become distressed soon after.

This is because their intestine is contracting on trapped wind from TWO feeds ago!

Why we need to burp babies MORE

If we burp babies more, we can prevent this discomfort and stop the unsettled behaviours.

If these symptoms sound like your little bundle of joy, then take a look at page 154 on recognising wind signs and page 164 on Dr Golly active burping technique. You'll soon see these problems melt away.

See
pg. 164

The Dr Golly active burping technique

When it comes to expelling wind correctly, the first thing to understand is that burping a baby is not as easy as it seems. Although we take it for granted, like farting, it's actually a highly complex, co-ordinated process.

As your baby feeds, they also suck in air. This air forms pockets or bubbles within the stomach, mixed in with the recent feed.

That bubble needs to separate from the milk, manoeuvre to the top of the stomach, then negotiate a valve and fly out the feeding tube.

It's a windy, difficult path to negotiate – **and it requires your help!**

Babies are not capable of burping themselves, because you just can't burp when you're lying flat on your back. This is why we need to 'burp' them, and why it's important to fully understand the process.

You need to burp your baby after every sucking period, whether the feed is taken as:

· two breasts
· a bottle in one go
· multiple sucks broken down.

> After EVERY period of sucking, whether two minutes or 20, that baby needs to be burped.

There is no magic number of burps, but usually 2–3 per sucking period is average. Some babies will burp twice, others eight times – and everything in between.

Signs that you're sufficiently burping your baby include:

· improved feed frequency
· absence of wind signs
· little to no settled/unsettled behaviour
· adequate weight gain.

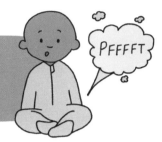

And remember, no matter how hilarious they are – **farts don't count as burping a baby!**

PFFFFT

So how do you go about burping a baby?

The first thing I want to address is one of the biggest myths out there:

Patting does nothing to help release wind!

Gentle patting or rubbing may settle/soothe a baby, and it is necessary to be settled and relaxed in order to expel wind, but patting does not equal burping!

TIP

The cadence of a pat should mimic a mother's heartbeat, not a sprinter's heart rate!

Mother's heartbeat:

Sprinter's heartbeat:

The number one secret to getting out that burp?

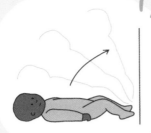

· ·

Simple: it's the transition from horizontal to vertical.

· ·

That's why parents often report their baby doing a burp after a nappy change, when they get picked up again. That's what we need to recreate.

The first burp is often the easiest, as the baby is moved from the feeding position, usually somewhat horizontal, to a vertical position.

The vertical position can vary according to what's comfortable for you.

Some options include:

On your lap using the V-grip: Use your thumb and index finger to support your baby's head, and keep their torso vertical. Remember not to let the baby hunch over, and make sure your fingers rest on their jawbone, to avoid putting any pressure on their neck and airway.

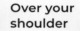

Over your shoulder

Against your chest

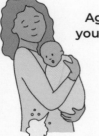

The important thing is that the baby is vertical.

Step 1:

Move the baby from the somewhat horizontal feeding position to a vertical position. Once vertical, keep your baby upright for a period of one minute.

Most babies will bring up their first burp. *Don't be concerned about a small, infrequent posset or spill of milk – these should not distract you from the important task at hand.*

After this first burp has erupted, **I want you to engage in a more ACTIVE burping process.**

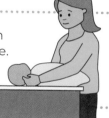

Here, you begin a 15-minute window of active burping, where you transition repeatedly from horizontal to vertical.

Step 2:

After one minute upright, lay your baby down on their back on a flat, hard and warm surface. Give your baby two minutes flat on their back, totally calm.

Step 3:

Lift them again to vertical, in a very slow transition.

Once they are upright, you can pat gently, or bounce as you walk, to help dislodge the wind pocket.

Keep your baby upright for one minute, then repeat the process.

Remember – two minutes down, one minute up. Repeat.

Usually, a 15-minute window is adequate to expel 2–3 burps.

You might repeat this process five, six or even ten times, depending on whether the wind signs have disappeared or how many burps your baby does per sucking period, on average.

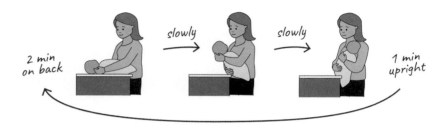

It's best to lay the baby on their back for the horizontal periods, but lying them on their stomach is also okay. This can be a nice way of fitting tummy time into the routine.

> **TIP**
>
> Carpet is best – avoid cold tiles or concrete, and ideally not a soft bed. If you're in public and don't want to use the floor, either put a towel on a table or, as a last resort, use your legs as the surface.

The importance of calm:

It's important for your baby to be completely calm when lying horizontally. This technique simply doesn't work if the baby is crying or straining from the wind. You can employ a number of different calming techniques to achieve two minutes of relaxed time to facilitate the next burp. These include rubbing the tummy, cycling the legs, singing and interacting with your baby, using a dummy briefly, patting and shushing, etc.

If your baby has become inconsolable and you can't achieve two minutes of calm, then move straight back to upright and try again later.

Also remember that a baby does not need to be awake to be burped! In some ways, it's easier to burp a sleeping baby because they're totally calm when lying flat. When your baby is fast asleep in their cot or bassinet, consider sitting them up in their sleep to try to get one last burp – ensuring an even longer sleep for everyone!

Active burping can be incorporated into your daily routine.

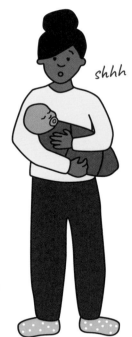

shhh

- Each nappy change is about two minutes lying flat – the perfect opportunity to burp.
- Lying down on a playmat? Another opportunity to burp.
- Applying moisturiser or cream to your baby, changing a onesie – these are all perfect opportunities to extract more burps.
- Tummy time provides another opportunity. You can even burp your baby in the bath using the exact same technique, just done in the water.

I know that many parents are reluctant to add another 'chore' to their feeding regimen, and long periods of active burping can add at least half an hour to each feed. But if the feeding frequency drops substantially because your baby is full of milk, not air, you'll soon see that the investment is worthwhile.

Some common questions about wind include:

(?) How do I manage burping when my baby is pulling off frequently?

The most common reason a baby pulls off after a few short sucks is due to the gastro-colic reflex. Trapped wind from the previous feed causes cramping in the colon as soon as the stomach starts to fill with milk from the current feed. While you may need to offer a quick burp each time your baby falls off the breast/bottle, it's important to understand that your baby is telling you they needed to burp more at the previous feed. Hopefully, when they are fully burped after this feed, you'll enter into a nice rhythm/cycle and see them sucking for longer periods of time at future feeds.

(?) Do I burp after each boob/bottle suck?

Yes, it's important to offer a burp after each side or at each break during a bottle-feed. The goal is to remove as much wind as possible to prevent discomfort in the coming hours. You don't have to offer the full 15 minutes of burping after each small break, but at least offer the full 15 minutes at the end of the feed.

(?) When are babies able to burp themselves?

You may need to burp your baby after feeds for many months, but babies do slowly get better at burping themselves the longer they spend upright. Also, as they take larger volumes of solids, the need for burping subsides.

(?) **Is there a certain number of burps we should aim for in each feeding session?**

There's no magic number of burps, as some are larger than others. That's why I like to devote a certain period of time to burping instead.

(?) **Do certain foods make breastfed babies more gassy?**

They certainly do! Foods that make adults gassy will also make babies gassy, such as broccoli or beans. Babies also sometimes struggle with spice, garlic or onion.

(?) **We only get a maximum of 1–2 burps per 15 minutes. If this happens within the first 5–10 minutes, can we stop there?**

The answer is yes – always respond to your baby. If they bring up all their wind in the first five minutes, there's no need to continue burping them for another ten minutes.

(?) **How important is the two minutes down, one minute up?**

Again, always respond to your baby. If you are achieving great burps with, say, one minute down and 30 seconds up, and your baby is showing no signs of discomfort from trapped wind, then that's great. If you're struggling to get burps, then the two minutes down, one minute up, for 15 minutes is really important.

(?) **Should the burp be loud and obvious?**

Your baby's burps might be loud or a small whimper. They are all bringing up air, but definitely not the same amount. It's important to burp your baby thoroughly using the active burping technique and to always watch your baby for signs of trapped wind. Remember, these may not be immediate, and you'll often see the associated unsettledness in the hours to come.

Is a little posset classed as a burp?

Yes – sometimes a big bubble of gas can carry a small posset above it. This is no problem (other than the mess!).

 My baby squirms and cries when horizontal after a feed, then vomits when picked up. Is there an alternative to having the baby lie fully flat?

Try keeping your baby upright for a few minutes before beginning the method. When flat, try cycling the legs, rubbing the tummy, interacting playfully or using a dummy, to try to get them as calm as possible. Remember, small possets don't matter, as long as baby is gaining good weight.

 My baby is so hard to burp, I'm lucky to get one in 15 minutes. It's making night wakings so much longer and I'm exhausted. Any advice?

Some babies are certainly harder to burp than others. If your active burping technique is right and you're devoting time to it after every feed, but still not getting more burps, I'd consider adding a colic mix to help the wind out more easily. See the colic section on page 174.

 What colic mix do you recommend?

As a paediatrician, I remain brand-agnostic when it comes to medicines, homeopathics and listed pharmaceuticals. There are a number of different products on the market, including simethicone, dicyclomine, belladonna, hyoscyamine and dozens more. It's important to discuss these with your child's doctor or paediatrician before administering any, due to potential side effects.

Can nipple shields increase the amount of air my baby swallows and make them more uncomfortable?

No. If your baby is attaching correctly around the shield this should not be any different to a bottle fed or breastfed baby – that is, they will all take in some air, and burping them after every sucking period is essential. I always recommend hand-expressing some milk into the top of the shield so that the first mouthful is milk, not air.

 Can I burp a sleeping baby?

I'm so glad you asked – the answer is YES! Many parents, particularly in the first four weeks, find their baby is showing tired signs before they have finished their active burping period. My advice here is to swaddle them and get them into the cot lying flat. If they are dozy or fully asleep you can still pick them up gently after a couple of minutes and get that last burp out. I often did the late-night feed. I'd put my baby down, go and brush my teeth and then come back to get that last burp ... it's sooo satisfying!

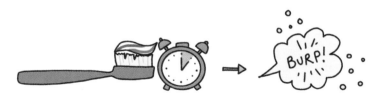

 Is the cot mattress too soft to use for the active burping technique?

For the full active burping technique, the cot mattress is not ideal – but if it's just for the last burp as your baby drifts off to sleep, then it's absolutely fine – see my notes above.

Hiccoughs

Hiccoughs ('hiccups' if you're using the Macquarie Dictionary) are a very strong sign that your baby has trapped wind.

All babies will hiccough – just like we adults do (every now and then). A lot of mums feel their baby hiccoughing in the womb. This is normal – there's no need to be distressed.

BUT if your baby:

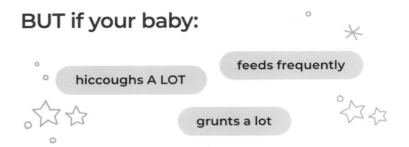

hiccoughs A LOT

feeds frequently

grunts a lot

These are strong signs that they need to be burped more, and that perhaps you need a more active burping method.

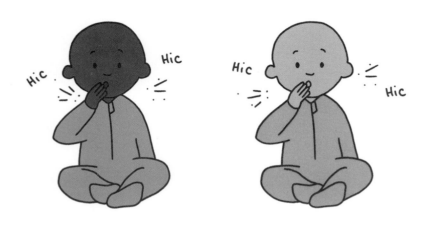

Some common questions about hiccoughs include:

(?) What if my baby starts hiccoughs as soon as I lie them down to burp them?

If your baby starts hiccoughing as soon as you start to burp them, this is just an indication that you need to do a really thorough burping that round. The hiccough shouldn't interrupt the burping method.

(?) Do hiccoughs expel trapped air? Do they count as a burp?

Unfortunately, while it feels like there is a lot of air coming up, a hiccough doesn't count as a burp. Again, it just means you have to burp more.

(?) How do I avoid hiccoughs in the first place?

Unfortunately there is no way to avoid hiccoughs. Babies are obligate nose breathers, so sometimes air just gets in. This doesn't mean you're doing anything wrong, it just means you have to help them get the air up.

COLIC

A note before you keep reading this chapter:

• •

Studies show colic impacts 10–20 per cent of babies, so statistics suggest most will be spared. Therefore, if you're preparing for birth, perhaps set this chapter aside for now, but if your baby is highly unsettled and crying more than you think they should, by all means dig deeper.

• •

Lots of the information in this chapter is available in my colic blog at **drgolly.com**. If you have friends who are navigating their way through early parenting with a colicky baby, please send them to the blog.

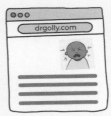

Parenting a colicky baby is unbelievably taxing, driving significantly higher rates of parental stress and post-natal depression. We need to support and empower everyone facing this challenge.

COLIC

What is colic?

Colic (also called 'infantile colic') is a word that describes a condition whereby a baby cries excessively. 'Excessively' is defined as more than three hours a day, for more than three days a week, for three weeks or more.

Colic most often becomes evident when a baby is 2–5 weeks old, and usually eases by the time the baby is 3–4 months old.

Common signs of infant colic:

Excessive crying

Knees pulling up, squirming during/after feeds

Fussy and irregular feeds, pulling off the breast or bottle frequently

General unsettledness and clingyness

Tendency to wake screaming

Visible discomfort and distress

Difficulty with burping, no matter how diligent you are

A LOT of farting

Strong preference to sleep upright, such as in the pram or carrier, and unhappiness when lying flat

Search 'colic', 'infantile colic' or 'purple crying' online and you'll mostly find two things:

1. ways to settle or distract an unsettled baby
2. reassuring messages that this torturous period will pass.

Incredibly, neither of these things addresses the underlying cause of colic, treating it instead as some kind of newborn rite of passage. It is important to appreciate that calling a baby 'colicky' does little more than attach an adjective to an unsettled baby without seeking to understand **why** they're unsettled.

This is absolutely wrong. Correcting the problem is the only solution, and **understanding the problem** is the crucial first step to correction. Colic is definitely NOT a period to 'suffer' through and survive.

> **Crying is normal, but excessive crying is not.**

Yes, babies cry. Yes, healthy babies cry. Yes, crying is a form of communication.

But excessive crying, frequent feeding, unsettled behaviour, short sleeps – these are all caused by something, and the key to eradicating colic is to understand what that something is.

Is purple crying the same as colic?

The terms 'colic' and 'purple crying' are often used interchangeably. It's important to remember that they are descriptive terms; they are not medical conditions or a disease.

The term 'purple crying' was originally coined to minimise shaken-baby syndrome by normalising the period of unsettled behaviour and infant crying that occurs between two weeks and four months.

It's actually an acronym:

Peak crying

Unexpected

Resistant to soothing

Pain-filled face

Long-lasting, and occurring in the

Evening.

Will babies grow out of colic?

Many babies will grow out of colic by the time they reach around four months of age, but four months of highly unsettled behaviour and crying is not something you should struggle through.

Find the cause, alleviate it – and enjoy a settled baby who sleeps!

What causes colic?

There are myriad reasons why babies are unsettled and cry excessively. By far the most common cause is inadequate burping.

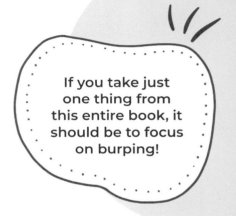

If you take just one thing from this entire book, it should be to focus on burping!

But colic can also be driven by:

hunger

illness

an immature gut unable to process some elements of milk

problems processing the volume of milk

quick letdowns (and guzzling babies)

poor attachment during feeding

eczema

intolerances

and everything in between

What to do if you think your baby has colic

Step 1: Burps, burps and more burps. Teach everyone in your family the Dr Golly active burping technique. Any time the baby isn't feeding, you can be burping them. Use the active burping technique for 15 minutes after each feeding period.

Step 2: Regular tummy time to strengthen their neck – the quicker they can crawl/sit up, the easier it will be to burp them and get that trapped wind out.

Step 3: If you're breastfeeding, be aware of your diet. If you're drinking/eating a lot of cow's milk, legumes, roughage, cured meats or fermented products, these could upset your baby. Remember, food that makes you gassy will make your baby gassy, too.

Step 4: If you're breastfeeding, be aware of caffeine in breastmilk, as this can cause unsettled behaviour. Absolutely enjoy this ritual – mums need their coffee – but be mindful of excess consumption.

Step 5: Check for all other causes that could be upsetting your baby, e.g. excess heat/cold, itchy clothing tag, uncontrolled eczema, overtiredness, undertiredness etc.

Step 6: Watch for food intolerances, which are not uncommon in breastfed babies. Mucus in the poo is a sign that your baby is intolerant to something.

Step 7: If you have completed the above steps and your baby is still uncomfortable/unsettled, it may be time to talk to your GP or paediatrician about a colic mix.

Remember, when it comes to colic/purple crying:

1. Medication should be your last step, not your first.

2. Colic mixes won't fix colic, but they will make your baby easier to burp, helping to expel trapped wind. Your family will need to be fastidious about burping.

3. If you think your baby has severe colic, you'll need to talk to your GP or paediatrician and work through what is happening.

4. There are lots of colic mixes out there – again, you'll need to see your GP or paediatrician about

   a) whether your baby needs pharmaceutical help

   b) which colic mix is the right one for your baby – be sure to discuss possible side effects, too.

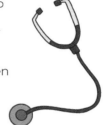

5. If you're talking to your GP or paediatrician, be open to the idea that colic may not be the problem. Always describe your baby's symptoms to your healthcare professional. It may help to track them in the notes app on your phone.

You need to resolve the cause of the unsettled behaviour, as:

- until you do, your baby is probably going to be unsettled due to the trapped wind/pain.

- colicky babies will rarely sleep in a cot, and have trouble linking sleep cycles.

 TIP

Allow for contact naps in the carrier or pram until you have the trapped wind pain or underlying condition under control.

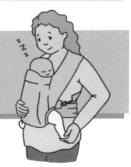

Caring for a colicky baby can be incredibly hard

• •

If you are struggling with a colicky baby, please know that you are not alone.

• •

If your baby won't stop crying and you're not coping, call a friend or family member for practical support.

The correlation between highly unsettled babies and perinatal mental health issues is almost one to one. All parents of unsettled babies are at an elevated risk of perinatal mental health issues. If you have previously struggled with anxiety or depression, then you are at an even higher risk.

If you need help, it is available. Seeking help early is the best thing you can do (see more on mental health on page 210).

See
pg. 210

A note to breastfeeding mothers trying to care for a colicky baby alone:

- If you are breastfeeding and you are a single parent, you need to find someone to support you until you resolve the trapped wind/unsettled behaviour. Please don't try to do it all yourself.
- If you are breastfeeding and your partner is away or works long hours, you need to find support.

TIP

If you're exhausted, you might be tempted by the idea of a holiday. Rather than taking a two-week vacation with an unsettled baby, I highly recommend you take two weeks at home taking care of each other and the baby, and working together to resolve whatever is driving the unsettled behaviour.

So much of my philosophy and practice is about protecting the breastfeeding mother. In nearly all cases, when the appropriate treatment is given and the non-breastfeeding parent spends significant time caring for both the baby and the breastfeeding mother, things improve significantly.

Colic does NOT mean you have to have an unhappy, unsettled baby who cries all the time. Numerous articles say there is no cure for colic and that some babies just cry – these are WRONG!

Colic has causes and solutions, we just need to find out what they are.

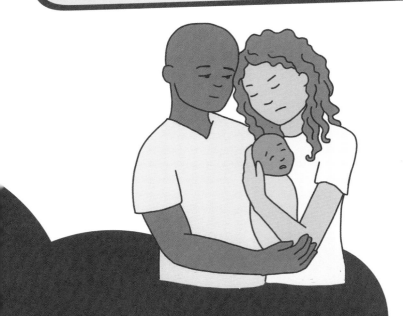

Vomit

Many parents get distressed when their baby brings up milk, but it's important not to panic. Not every spill of milk is a true vomit, and not all refluxed milk means your baby has reflux.

There are generally four types of 'vomit' that need to be defined.

 Bright green vomit of any volume can also be a sign of obstruction and requires urgent medical attention.

 1. **First is a small, effortless ejection of milk – this is known as a posset.** These cause no distress, no weight loss, no issues at all.

Possets occur in almost half of all babies, usually beginning before two months of age and peaking at four months.

Happy spitters

Some babies will posset after every feed – sometimes even hours after a feed has concluded. These babies are often described as 'happy spitters' and, despite the inconvenience to the parent, the possets are of no concern. The positive to having 'happy spitters' is that they tend to bring wind up very easily, and they are often the most settled babies in town!

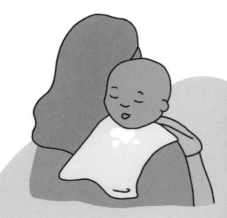

Your baby's tummy is like a balloon

When a baby feeds, their stomach becomes overstretched, especially if it is full of milk and wind. Think of a full water balloon, before you tie a knot at the top. Like a stretched balloon, any muscle in the body wants to return to its original size, and will therefore rebound, much as an untied balloon deflates rapidly when released.

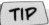

As the stomach tries to return to its original size, this can often result in a column of milk rising up the oesophagus (feeding tube) and spilling out. These are called 'possets'.

> **TIP**
>
> By deflating the stomach with more burping, we can reduce the chance of that rising column of milk, and actually reduce possets. (See page 162 for more.)

2. **The second type of vomit *is* a vomit.** This is an ejection of the stomach contents, involving retching/gagging and the movement of other muscles, like the shoulders lifting up. This will empty the stomach and, yes, this milk needs to be replaced. Large vomits occurring infrequently are not problematic, but recurrent vomiting needs to be investigated.

3. **Projectile vomit.** This is caused by an obstructed stomach, most commonly caused by pyloric stenosis (an uncommon condition in infants that blocks food from entering the small intestine). This is unmissable – the vomit will hit the ceiling or the wall behind you, and worsens quickly. Projectile vomiting is a medical emergency.

4. **True reflux.** Gastro-oesophageal reflux disease is an uncommon condition, in which frequent milk reflux leads to feed refusal, poor growth, bloody vomits, irritability and a chronic cough. This needs to be checked by a doctor.

Reflux

Reflux is not as common as most people think.

Many people incorrectly refer to possets as reflux, or even worse: silent reflux. It is important not to medicate a baby for reflux when it is *not* the cause of their unsettled behaviour.

Small spills of milk by a happy, growing baby are completely normal. They don't cause unsettledness. A wonderful 2006 study led by Australian paediatricians showed no link between 'spills' and crying time or back-arching.

Despite this, reflux has become the go-to, rapid explainer of unsettled behaviour, becoming synonymous with colic.

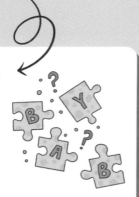

Dismissing unsettled behaviour as reflux is problematic for two reasons:

1. The true cause of that baby's unsettled behaviour is being missed.

2. The medication usually prescribed for reflux is not without side-effects.

True reflux has very serious symptoms.

True gastro-oesophageal reflux disease is not common. Babies who suffer from true reflux have very specific symptoms, including weight loss, severe feeding difficulties and bloody vomit.

Anti-reflux medications

Between 2000 and 2003 there was a 400 per cent increase in the prescribing of anti-reflux medication, yet no reduction in the incidence of colic. This speaks volumes about the true incidence of reflux.

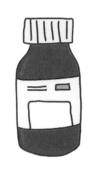

Anti-reflux medications have risks and very real long-term side effects, including respiratory and gastrointestinal infections, as well as poor bone health.

We know that the two most commonly prescribed groups of medicines (H2 receptor antagonists and proton pump inhibitors) had no effect when compared with a placebo medicine.

An incorrect diagnosis of reflux leads to the prescribing of unnecessary medications and an undesirable spiral of 'medicalisation', which we need to avoid.

Silent reflux is a myth

Reflux is so overdiagnosed that when milk spillage doesn't occur, unsettled behaviour is referred to as *silent reflux*. This is incorrect and potentially dangerous, sadly leading to treatment which only worsens the original, undiagnosed problem.

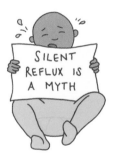

Silent reflux is a myth – it simply does not exist.
Never let your baby's unsettled behaviour be dismissed as silent reflux. The treatments can be harmful, and often they will worsen colic.

Find your rhythm, not routine

Many parents crave the predictability of a routine. This is understandable: the benefits are clear.

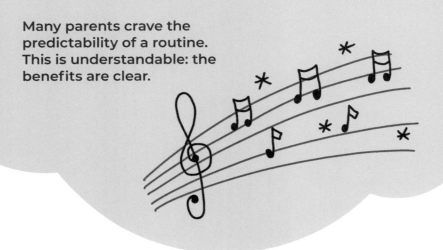

However, seeking to establish one too early will only be met with disappointment. It's important to ensure your expectations are realistic. I don't recommend establishing a routine until your baby is roughly six weeks (corrected) and 5–6 kilograms, this is to provide ample time for parent–baby bonding and showing your baby that you are responsive to their needs.

We want our babies to be nice and robust and with established breastmilk supply (if you're breastfeeding) before we move into a routine.

There's still plenty you can do in the first four weeks of life, though!

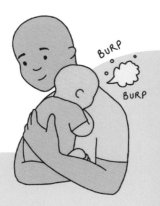

You may like to work towards a gentle daily rhythm.

Most babies will be feeding in 3–4 hour cycles by 3–6 weeks, potentially with a longer stretch overnight. This passage is deliberately vague, as there's so much variability in what's 'normal'!

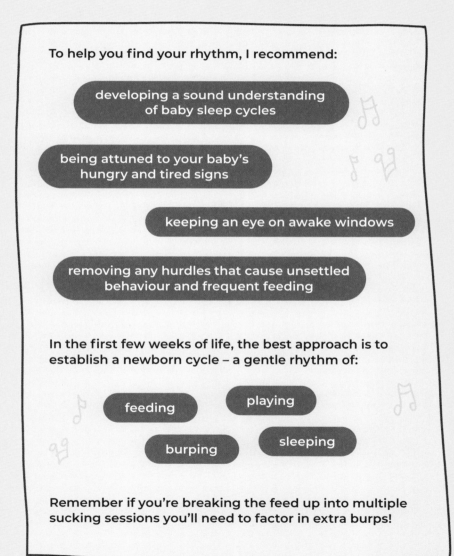

To help you find your rhythm, I recommend:

developing a sound understanding of baby sleep cycles

being attuned to your baby's hungry and tired signs

keeping an eye on awake windows

removing any hurdles that cause unsettled behaviour and frequent feeding

In the first few weeks of life, the best approach is to establish a newborn cycle – a gentle rhythm of:

feeding

playing

burping

sleeping

Remember if you're breaking the feed up into multiple sucking sessions you'll need to factor in extra burps!

This newborn cycle provides the crucial foundation for a more predictable routine from six weeks of age, setting your entire family up for sleeping through the night – earlier than most people think possible!

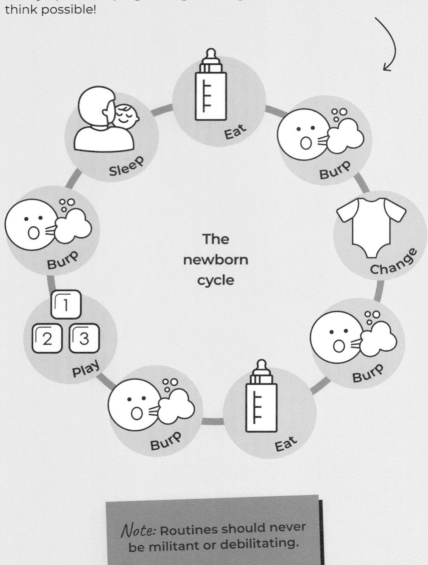

The newborn cycle

Eat · Burp · Change · Burp · Eat · Burp · Play · Burp · Sleep

Note: Routines should never be militant or debilitating.

Even after six weeks, routines should never be followed with militant precision. You should still be attuned and responsive to your baby's tired or hungry signs (and your own schedule) and remain flexible.

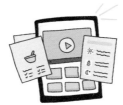

My online programs include suggested routines for six weeks and beyond. These are intentionally flexible – all times include 30 minutes of 'give or take' during the day or night, with lots of options to adapt the routine when you're on the go or out and about.

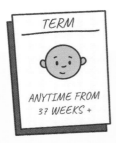

TERM

ANYTIME FROM 37 WEEKS +

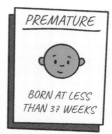

PREMATURE

BORN AT LESS THAN 37 WEEKS

A note on premature babies:
A 'term' birth is considered anytime from 37 weeks onwards. A baby born at less than 37 weeks is considered premature. When considering a rhythm or routine for your baby, all targets (sleep, weight, length, head circumference, development targets) need to be based on your baby's **corrected age.** This means the age they would be, had they arrived on their due date of 40 weeks. This correction should be continued for at least six months when considering targets.

Awake windows

Newborns are still adjusting to the world around them, and can only handle a very short period of awake time before they begin to show signs of tiredness and need to be settled to sleep.

In the first four weeks they may only have an hour of awake time, sometimes less. This can be surprising for many new parents.

For most newborns, this is just enough time for a feed, nappy change and active burping.

Watch closely for tired signs as your baby approaches the end of their awake window, and settle your baby to sleep within ten minutes of recognising these signs, to ensure they don't become overtired. See page 152 for more on signs of tiredness.

See pg. 152

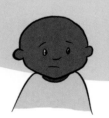
I'm getting tired

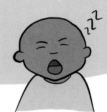
I'm ready for bed

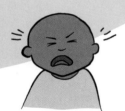
I'm overtired

Is your baby falling asleep while feeding?

It can be difficult to keep your baby awake during a feed in those first few weeks of life. Often they're so comfortable, warm and tired from feeding that falling asleep is inevitable. While this is very normal, it can also be frustrating.

To help keep your newborn awake during a feed:

- Strip your baby down to just their nappy and enjoy skin-to-skin contact. This helps stimulate the natural instinct to find the breast and feed.

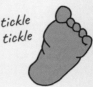

tickle
tickle

- Stimulate your baby gently during the feed by tickling their feet, stroking their back, blowing on their face, etc.

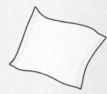

- Keep a damp, cool face washer next to you and gently dab your baby's forehead if they begin to fall asleep.

- Compress your breasts – this can help stimulate the flow of milk when it has slowed down, especially if your baby is tiring.

- Watch your baby for early feeding cues (when they're starting to be hungry), and feed before they exhibit late cues (distressed crying – when they're ravenous), as by this stage your baby will have exerted a lot of energy and may not sustain a longer feed.

- Offer a burp. Trapped air will make your baby think they are full, so getting rid of this will allow them to feed for longer.

- Change feeding positions to help wake them up if they're starting to get sleepy.

- During the day, feed them in a brightly lit room, and don't be scared to turn on the TV or music.

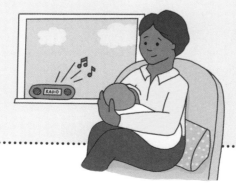

Sleep cycles

All humans progress through a cycle during sleep. This sees a slow transition from light to heavy sleep and back again.

A baby's sleep cycle in the first four weeks is approximately 45 minutes, roughly half that of an adult (90 minutes).

40–45 min
Light sleep, easy to wake up

0–10 min
Starting to fall asleep

Baby's sleep cycle every 45 minutes

30–40 min
Coming out of heavy sleep

10–20 min
Getting deeper into sleep

20–30 min
Heavily asleep

For neonates (babies in their first month of life) there are three stages of sleep:

 REM (rapid eye movement, active) sleep

 Non-REM (deep) sleep

 Transitional sleep (a combination of both active and deep).

Deep sleep makes up half of a newborn's total sleep time, which is why they are often able to sleep through noise, light, etc.

 With a single sleep cycle being 40–45 minutes long, it's important that we help our babies 'stitch' together individual sleep cycles to achieve adequate total sleep time.

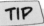

When linking sleep cycles, it's important to manage your own expectations. You may have a baby who does this perfectly for the first 2–3 weeks and then 'wakes up' and can't do it anymore. This is very common, so don't panic. Trust the process – laying all the correct foundations is going to pay off. Linking sleep cycles is a learned skill for babies, and some won't be developmentally able to do this until they are 4–5 months old.

Persistence, patience and consistency are key.

From four months onwards, sleep development progresses and babies mature to a more adult-style sleep architecture. These cycles slowly get longer, until they match adult lengths, at around three years of age.

Top tips for linking sleep cycles

Tip 1:
A conducive room environment.

This is where an ideal sleep environment (see pages 120–126) is crucial.

A dark room with white noise playing will help your baby fall back to sleep and transition through to the next sleep cycle.

Tip 2:
Put your baby to sleep in the same spot they will wake up.

Babies should ideally be put down to sleep in the same place they will wake up.

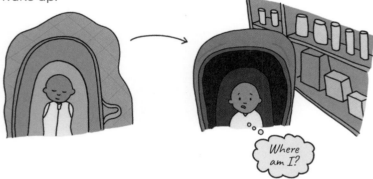

Just imagine if you fell asleep somewhere and woke up somewhere completely different. You'd most likely wake suddenly, and be frightened and unable to settle. Babies are exactly the same. For this reason, try not to rock your baby to sleep in your arms.

Tip 3:
Put them to bed sleepy, not asleep.

Aim to put your baby in their cot/bassinet while they're sleepy, but not yet asleep.

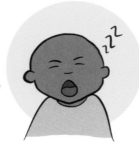

We want them to settle to sleep by themselves, without needing to be rocked or fed to sleep. This means the way they fall asleep is the way they wake up – and there will be no surprise.

Tip 4:

Make sure they have enough sleep debt.

If your baby is waking after a single sleep cycle and is unable to resettle, this could be because they have not accumulated enough sleep debt.

Increasing their awake time by 5–15 minutes can sometimes be helpful.

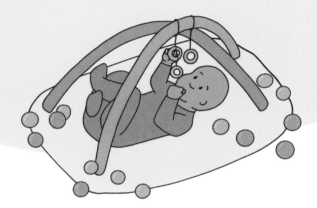

Tip 5:

If they wake after 45 minutes, you can continue their sleep upright in the carrier.

Babies love being close to us, and if they are unsettled, being upright can often help.

If a baby stirs and doesn't resettle (try not to jump in too early), you can pop them in the carrier to ensure they get a nice long stretch of sleep. This will help avoid overtiredness and catnapping.

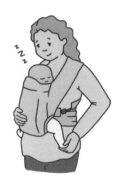

Tip 6:

Remove all other hurdles that could be causing them to wake and not resettle after a cycle.

You can see the full list of hurdles on page 157.

Circadian rhythm

Circadian rhythm refers to the body's 24-hour cycle.

Although babies wake and sleep multiple times throughout the day, they still learn to tell the difference between night and day.

This helps to:

· elongate their night sleeps
· coincide their sleep with your sleep patterns
· cluster their feeds and wakefulness to the daytime.

How to encourage a good circadian rhythm in your baby

Tip 1:
Expose children to the busyness of a day routine and the calm of night-time.

DAY	NIGHT
Expose them to sunlight.	Ensure lighting is minimal.
Ensure they hear noises.	Ensure sounds are quiet and soothing.
Ensure they feel movement.	Try a warm, relaxing bath to create a lovely evening sleep association.

Tip 2:

Engage in a repetitive rhythm as soon as possible.

This will help to drive the establishment of a routine.

It's difficult to alter circadian rhythms, as you may have experienced when travelling across time zones and feeling jet lagged, or when working a night shift.

Tip 3:

Breastfeed in the evening and through the night (where possible).

This increases baby's intake of tryptophan, which is contained in breastmilk and encourages the production of melatonin.

Melatonin is our natural sleep hormone.

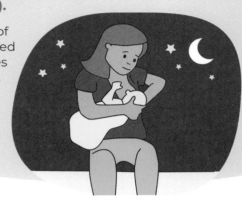

Tip 4:

Avoid excessive stimulation overnight.

Keep feeds quiet and calm, and make sure the room is dimly lit to encourage your baby to learn the difference between night and day.

Doing this will maximise the chances of dropping overnight feeds, instead of your baby having long daytime sleeps and cluster feeding in the evening.

Tip 5:

Don't pick your baby up if they are making sounds/movements but remain asleep.

Babies can be very active and noisy throughout their sleeps. This usually means they're cycling through non-REM sleep.

Be mindful not to stimulate them to wake when they are capable of returning to deep sleep by themselves.

Tummy time

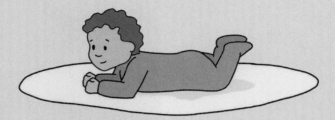

Tummy time happens when your baby lies on their tummy with weight on their forearms. Tummy time builds head, neck and upper body strength.

• •

It's wonderful for promoting gross motor development, interacting with your baby and enjoying baby time without a focus on feeding or burping.

• •

The recent phenomenon of tummy time

Historically, sudden infant death syndrome (SIDS) rates were once disturbingly high. When the American Academy of Pediatrics launched their Back-to-Sleep campaign in 1994, which promoted sleeping babies on their backs, this saw a phenomenal 50 per cent reduction in SIDS episodes almost immediately.

While this is undoubtedly successful and should never be challenged, placing children on their backs resulted in some unwanted side effects, too.

1. **Positional plagiocephaly (flat head syndrome).** See more on page 148.

2. **Colic.** Babies generally sleep better on their stomachs, as they are less bothered by wind in this position, and more capable of burping independently. See more on page 174.

3. **Delayed gross motor development** due to less time spent on their stomachs, which means less time pushing up, strengthening their back, shoulder and neck muscles. This delays the strength and co-ordination required for sitting, standing, etc. Studies have found that back sleepers eventually develop their motor skills just fine and these discrepancies don't last.

Tummy time now exists to alleviate these three side effects.

Some babies, however, strongly dislike lying on their stomachs. If this is the case with your baby, don't feel the need to force it. Many parents get really stressed about tummy time – and I urge you not to. Plenty of babies spend very minimal time on their stomachs and still go on to develop perfectly normally.

> In a 2008 study, researchers reported that babies who were given more awake tummy time rolled and crawled earlier than those who were given less, but that they didn't learn to sit or walk, or develop other motor skills, any sooner.

There are certainly demonstrable benefits to promoting tummy time beyond gross motor development. Researchers also found ties between gross motor development and cognitive skill acquisition – which suggests that tummy time may also make kids smarter. This is probably because infants who are able to sit up have a more advanced understanding of the three-dimensional nature of objects, perhaps in part because when they can sit comfortably, they can more easily explore and inspect their toys.

Babies who spend more time crawling and walking, regardless of their age, also have better spatial memory skills. A 2014 study found that babies often learn to walk right before they learn language skills – so if they learn to walk earlier, they might talk earlier too. It's important not to overthink this, though. How quickly a child progresses developmentally has no impact on their long-term abilities.

So, yes, tummy time is good – but you don't need to overly fret about it.

How long should my baby do tummy time for?

Keep in mind that just a minute or two – even just 30 seconds – of tummy time will add up if you do it regularly. If your baby really hates it, try placing them on your chest/tummy instead of on the floor.

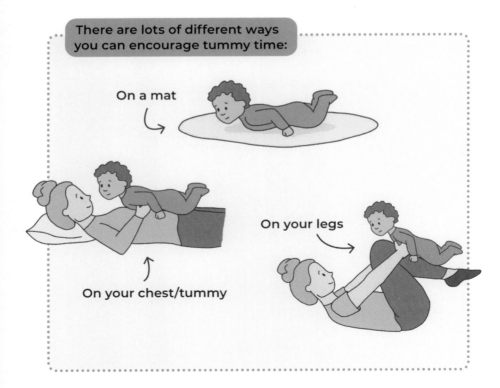

There are lots of different ways you can encourage tummy time:

On a mat

On your chest/tummy

On your legs

Development in the first month of life

Newborn reflexes

In the first month of life, almost all of a baby's abilities are still due to newborn reflexes:

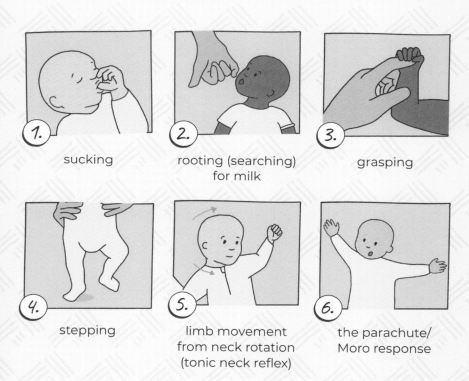

1. sucking

2. rooting (searching) for milk

3. grasping

4. stepping

5. limb movement from neck rotation (tonic neck reflex)

6. the parachute/ Moro response

This means that most of a newborn baby's movements are not intentionally performed.

Vision

Vision is one of the fastest developing systems of the body. By four weeks of age, you will notice your baby begins to focus on your eyes, will recognise their parents' faces and be able to briefly track movement.

At birth, babies are extremely short-sighted and can only really see the difference between light and dark. This is the reason why most mothers notice their nipples becoming darker during pregnancy – to help their newborn more easily identify the food source!

You'll notice that many newborn baby books are composed of black and white silhouettes, for this reason.

With time, the baby's depth of vision improves, and by one month, they can start to focus on your face. Many parents note a cross-eyed appearance; this is because the eyes are not yet binocular, meaning they don't yet work in unison. In most cases, this will rapidly normalise.

Note: If one eye is fixed sideways, this should be reviewed by an ophthalmologist (eye specialist).

Protecting your newborn's hearing

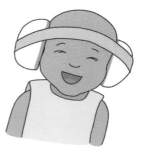

This advice goes far beyond the first four weeks and is good to keep in mind for the first years of life. If you're heading somewhere noisy, protective earmuffs are highly recommended for little ears.

Infants and young children are more sensitive to loud noises than adults are because the ear canal is smaller in children, and the sound pressure that is generated in the ears is greater compared to adults. In other words, loud sounds are even louder for kids.

Most audiologists will recommend hearing protection for sounds louder than 85 decibels, and government guidelines mandate that employees not be exposed to noise of 85 decibels or louder for longer than eight hours. But it's not a hard line. Consistent sounds over, say, 80 decibels could also be damaging.

It is important to limit both the intensity and duration of noise.

We also want to ensure that as our babies grow, we don't make our children anxious about noise.

There are apps on your phone that can measure the decibel level, but as a general guide:

· Comfortable noise levels are 0–60 dB, which would be things like conversational speech, nature sounds, or noise in your bedroom or living room.

· Loud noise levels are 60–90 dB, which are things like street traffic, heavy trucks or a live concert.

· Painful noise levels are anything above 90 dB and would include things like alarms, jackhammers or a jet engine.

Earplugs are not recommended for infants, toddlers or very young children, as they are small enough to present a choking hazard. Older children can use ear putty or appropriate-sized ear plugs to protect hearing.

What can I do to promote my baby's development?

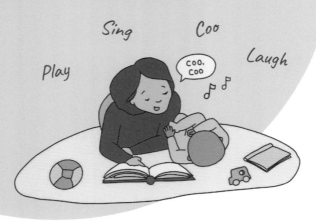

Be present and enjoy your time together. Put your phone away. A baby's interactions with their parents are the greatest drivers of development.

Read books and sing frequently – your baby recognises familiar voices.

A note on 'cooing': One of a baby's first forms of communication involves high-pitched nonsensical babble. This is your baby's first attempt at communicating verbally with you. Just as you'd never ignore someone speaking directly to you, you should not ignore this either! Don't respond with words – respond with the exact, high-pitched coo sound that your baby offers you.

Rapidly, you'll find a genuine two-way conversation occurring. This is laying incredible foundations for powerful language and communication skills. It's also hysterical, fun and one of life's greatest pleasures.

Playfully mimicking or returning infant babbling lets the child know that they can communicate, and this knowledge helps the infant learn the complex sounds that make up speech.

When should I be concerned about my baby's general development?

- If your baby is not showing signs of developmental progression, or is losing previously acquired skills.

- If they are not moving their arms or legs, especially if they are only moving one side or showing a hand preference.

- If they are not responding to your smile, face or voice.

- If your baby is demonstrating excessive sleepiness or lethargy.

Generally speaking, a parent's instincts are seldom misguided. If you are concerned about your baby's development, get this checked. Seeking help early can provide significant reassurance if everything is tracking along beautifully. And if there are any concerns, identifying problems early maximises the potential for intervention.

Myth-busting 'leaps'

Many parents will have heard of the publication
***The Wonder Weeks*. This is the English version**
of a Dutch book released in 1992, which draws
on data dating back to Jane Goodall's experience
observing chimpanzees in the 1970s.

The original authors of *The Wonder Weeks* were developmental psychologist and ethologist Frans Plooij and his wife, physical anthropologist Hetty van de Rijt, who studied 15 babies to produce the 'leap' thesis.

If you dig deeper into the original findings, you'll realise there is a lot of controversy surrounding the research and it has been dismissed by most professionals in the field.

SCHOLARLY SCANDAL

- In the early 2000s, researchers from universities in Spain, England and Sweden did try to replicate the 1992 results in three different studies. With a total of just 66 babies, the numbers aren't substantial, nor the research methods vigorous enough, to support an entire hypothesis.

- Frans Plooij's PhD student Carolina De Weerth attempted to replicate the original study with the biggest cohort of babies, but was unable to find evidence of the leaps.

- Plooij was vocal in criticising his student's study, and fought to keep it from being published.

- The paper was eventually published in 2011, and the controversy ultimately led Plooij to lose his place in academia.

- Despite this, 'Wonder Week' products still exist – with no caveats to the shortcomings of the findings.

Leaping to conclusions

The term 'developmental leaps' refers to ten predictable developmental phases that supposedly coincide with unsettled behaviour and sleep regression in babies. These leaps are said to occur at exactly the same time for every baby.

Sounds lovely, predictable and ordered, right? This idea provides solace to parents who are trying to understand why their child is unsettled, and gives them licence to 'ride it out' until the leap is finished.

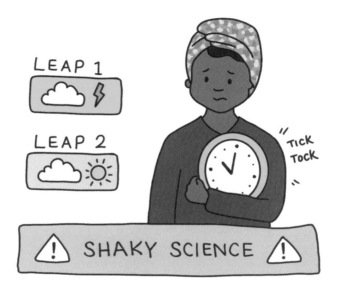

Unfortunately, this is based on very shaky science, and dismissed by most current paediatric psychologists and paediatricians in the field.

More importantly, these so-called leaps offer no solutions to what is driving unsettled behaviour, meaning the real problem can go unaddressed. This makes them potentially dangerous, and fundamentally unfair to both babies and parents.

Don't ever dismiss unsettled behaviour as a developmental leap.

Baby and child development occurs on a continuum

If you're a parent with an unsettled baby, at some point someone will surely tell you, *'Don't worry, it's just a leap.'* But as we just learned, **it's NOT a leap**, because leaps don't exist in a predictable, orderly and timed fashion.

Baby and child development is a fluid process. It occurs at different times and at different rates for every child.

There are countless variables and influences that affect the rate of child development, so to distil this complex, astonishing process into ten conveniently discrete stages that occur at exactly the same age in every child is simply misleading.

I would never want a parent to dismiss unsettled behaviour as 'just another leap' while potentially missing a treatable cause of poor feeding or reduced sleep.

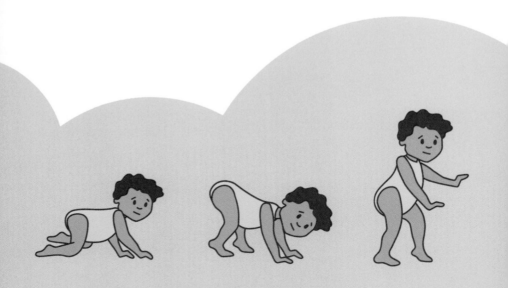

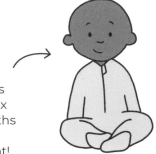

You would never state that a baby learns to sit independently the day they turn six months of age. It can occur at five months or at eight months. And this is an easily demonstrable gross motor development!

So how can you possibly predict complex neurological breakthroughs, in a newborn, down to the day?

There is one positive about the program, though: it encourages parents to interact with their babies and further drive their development.

However, simply playing with your child will achieve exactly the same thing. Development happens organically through play, through interaction, through talking and singing and with normal love and affection.

Doctor's orders: Do not engage with apps, books or social media accounts that talk about leaps. Instead, think of development as a fluid process. Trust your parental instincts, make time for tummy time, play, talk, sing and read to your baby, and start looking for the true cause of your child's unsettled behaviour.

Parents and mental health

For many parents, having a new baby is a time of happiness and joy. However, even normal adjustment to parenting can bring a range of emotions. Baby Blues, postnatal depression (PND), postnatal anxiety (PNA) and other mental illnesses can all occur after birth and at any time throughout parenthood.

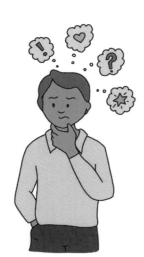

Being informed and knowing when to seek help are the keys to keeping yourself well.

In this section we'll talk through what is normal and what is:

1. postnatal depression (PND)
2. postnatal anxiety (PNA)
3. another mental illness.

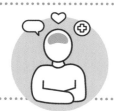

Note: As mentioned at the start of this book, if you have previously experienced anxiety or depression, having a proactive mental health plan ready to go as part of your postpartum preparation is one of the best things you can do.

Normal mental health adjustment

Joy, happiness, apprehension and some degree of worry are all normal for new parents. Such feelings may increase over the first few weeks.

For the birthing mother, you may be tired following the birth, in pain or busy trying to cope with your changing body and establish breastfeeding.

Many non-birthing parents feel helpless and excluded from breastfeeding, and may struggle to find a connection with their newborn and their partner.

For both parents, particularly in the first four weeks, sleep deprivation is an unavoidable aspect of parenthood. Even the most settled babies will feed every 3–4 hours (day and night).

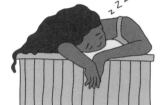

Both parents need time to adjust and learn how to be parents, and your baby needs time to adjust and learn how to be a baby.

Remember: When your baby is one week old, you are a one-week-old parent.

Everything is going to be a perfectly chaotic mess. Go easy on yourself, and be kind to yourself and each other as you all learn together.

The Baby Blues

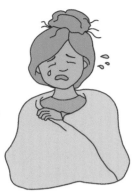

Between 80 and 85 per cent of women experience the Baby Blues after birth. This generally peaks at around days 3–5, and usually settles within a few days, but sometimes up to two weeks.

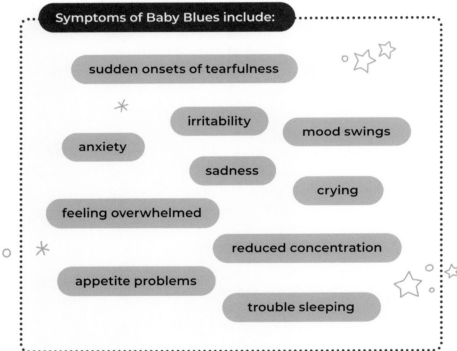

Symptoms of Baby Blues include:

sudden onsets of tearfulness

irritability

mood swings

anxiety

sadness

crying

feeling overwhelmed

reduced concentration

appetite problems

trouble sleeping

When might it not be the Baby Blues?

If the Baby Blues persist beyond two weeks, or if you develop mood changes after the first few weeks and your ability to function is affected, it is possible you may be developing postnatal depression (PND), postnatal anxiety (PNA) or another illness.

Postnatal depression, anxiety and psychosis

Postnatal depression (PND) affects up to one in five mums and up to one in ten dads after birth. Symptoms last longer than two weeks, and your ability to function is impaired.

Common symptoms of PND include:

- a numb, sad or low mood
- excessive crying
- a loss of interest in enjoyable activities, including those with your baby
- difficulty sleeping (not due to your baby waking) or excessive sleeping
- loss or increased appetite and/or weight loss or gain.

Postnatal anxiety (PNA) is thought to be more common than PND. Research has found that, as with PND, one in five women experience at least one type of anxiety disorder during pregnancy or postpartum.

PNA symptoms vary, but include:

- anxiety, fear or worry that is difficult to control, such as about your baby's health, sleeping or feeding
- feeling irritable, tense, restless, on edge
- increased heart rate or breathing, nausea or the shakes
- difficulty falling asleep at night (including when your baby is asleep)
- excessive checking on your baby.

Depression and anxiety symptoms often occur together.

A small proportion of mothers (1–2 per 1000 births) are affected by the rare but serious illness of postpartum psychosis (PPP). If you experience any of the following symptoms, it is important to seek help as soon as possible:

- elevated, irritable or up and down moods
- increased or racing thoughts
- increased talking
- a reduced need for sleep
- an increase in activity
- disorganisation
- hearing voices and/or having false belief or delusions
- thoughts of harming yourself or your baby.

Factors that may increase your risk of PND, PNA or PPP include:

- a past history of depression, anxiety or bipolar disorder
- a family history of mental illness, especially PPP, bipolar disorder or other mental illness related to childbirth
- traumatic birth experience
- a lack of support, including from your partner
- stressful life events, e.g. moving, renovating, changing jobs, a loss of job, the death of a loved one.

If you think you are suffering from:

- postnatal depression
- postnatal anxiety
- postpartum psychosis
- or if you have thoughts of harm to yourself or your baby.

REMEMBER:

1. Seeking help is essential
2. Help is available.

With the right care, postnatal depression, postnatal anxiety and postpartum psychosis can be treated and you can recover.

Seeking help can be challenging

The process of seeking help can sometimes appear daunting, if you don't know where to start. But one in five mums and one in ten dads will need help along the way. There is nothing shameful about seeking help and you are not a bad parent – quite the contrary, seeking help means you are doing exactly what you need to do to be the best parent for your baby.

How to go about seeking help

Speak to your partner, a family member or a friend so that they can support you to contact your GP, mental health professional or the Crisis Assessment and Treatment Team for your area.

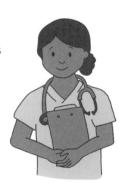

Speak to your obstetrician, maternal child health nurse, GP or mental health practitioner. They may refer you to a **perinatal psychiatrist or psychologist.**

You've got this!

Whether you're prepping for a new arrival or your baby is already here, remember:

(1.) When it comes to postpartum planning and care:

- Focus on protecting the breastfeeding mother.
- Never be afraid to ask for help and support.
- Whatever your current plan is for support, double it and you'll probably come close to what you need.

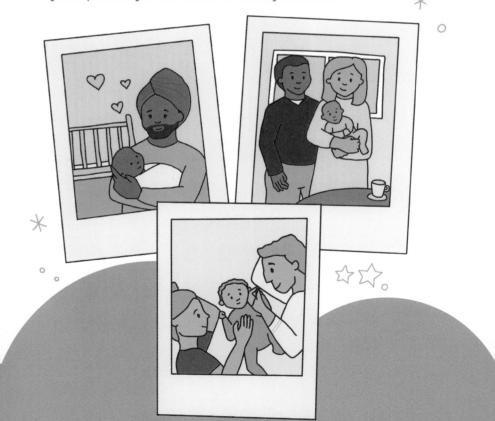

Babies drink more than milk.

- They drink all our emotions: good, bad and everything in between.
- When in doubt, take a big breath in, relax your shoulders, wiggle your bum and blow out any anxious, angry or negative energy.
- Hold your baby with confidence that whatever is happening, you'll work through it.

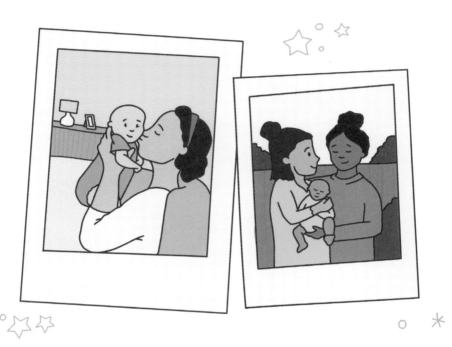

AND MOST IMPORTANTLY ...

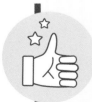

It's within you to do this. Your innate parental instincts are primal and powerful – trust them.

Author acknowledgements

Thank you to everyone who has contributed and reviewed the book. To the publishing and editing team at Hardie Grant Children's Publishing – what an extraordinary group you are. Alannah – you've been on this journey every step of the way and to say that none of this would be possible without you is an understatement. To Cora – you have brought this book and everything else I do to life across mediums, you are a wonder. To Alex, Jill and Adaobi – your collective expertise has been invaluable.

To the thousands of families who have joined the Dr Golly Sleep Program and follow me across platforms, I thank you for your ongoing support. I am so thrilled to be building an incredible community of families around the world.

 To learn more about the **Dr Golly Sleep Programs** please head to **drgolly.com**

 Follow me **@drgolly**

 Listen to my podcast **Dr Golly & The Experts**

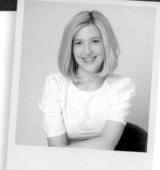

Cora Muccitelli
Illustrator

Cora is an illustrator and art director/ designer based in Surrey, UK. With nearly two decades of design experience, this is her first illustrated book – a childhood aspiration since she first started drawing. Cora has two beautiful boys who bring her endless joy and is very grateful to have had Dr Golly's wisdom guiding her through motherhood. Working with the brand since inception, she has loved bringing his philosophy of empowering parents to life across all channels.